HEALING BERRIES

HEALING
BERRIES

50 WONDERFUL BERRIES, AND HOW TO USE THEM
IN HEALTH-GIVING FOODS AND DRINKS

KIRSTEN HARTVIG

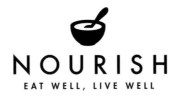

NOURISH
EAT WELL, LIVE WELL

To birds, for spreading joy and seeds

Healing Berries
Kirsten Hartvig

First published in the UK and USA in 2016 by
Nourish, an imprint of Watkins Media Limited
19 Cecil Court
London WC2N 4EZ

enquiries@nourishbooks.com

Editors: Carolyn Ryden, Elinor Brett, Rebecca Woods
Designers: Jade Wheaton, Suzanne Tuhrim, Clare Thorpe

A CIP record for this book is available from the British Library

ISBN: 9781848991552

1 3 5 7 9 10 8 6 4 2

Typeset in Futura
Colour reproduction by XY Digital
Printed in China

PLEASE NOTE
The nutritional and calorie information is based upon the ingredients listed for each recipe,
not for any alternative ingredients or additional serving suggestions.

MEASUREMENTS
Do not mix metric and imperial measurements.
1 tsp = 5ml   1 tbsp = 15ml   1 cup = 240ml

DISCLAIMER
The information in this book is intended to be helpful and informative. It is not meant to replace professional
medical advice, and should be used at the reader's discretion. While every care has been taken in compiling
the recipes for this book, Watkins Media Limited, or any other persons who have been involved in working
on this publication, cannot accept responsibility for any errors or omissions, inadvertent or not, that may be
found in the recipes or text, nor for any problems that may arise as a result of preparing one of these recipes.
If you are pregnant or breastfeeding or have any special dietary requirements or medical conditions,
it is advisable to consult a medical professional before following any of the recipes contained in this book.
Some foraged ingredients such as berries can be fatally poisonous. Neither the publisher nor the authors can
take any responsibility for any illness or other unintended consequences resulting from following any of the
advice or suggestions in this book.

CONTENTS

INTRODUCTION

This book describes 50 different berries: where to find them, how to prepare and use them, and how they can benefit health. It is written to enable culinary explorers, as well as foragers, campers and backpackers, to identify and use berries at home and away, and it includes more than 100 delicious recipes that feature berries. I have written this book in the belief that nature provides for all – wildlife and human beings – as long as we are not too greedy and do not destroy the plants that grow the berries, nor the habitats that support them. When we remember to share, always leaving something behind as seed for the next generation, we discover that abundance is truly nature's way.

Writing *Healing Berries* has taken more than two years, during which time my family and I have travelled many miles and tested myriad menus featuring berries as the main ingredient. The hunt for more elusive wild berries took us to many remote and beautiful places, and we quickly learnt the importance of good walking boots, long-sleeved shirts, tear-proof long trousers and lightweight materials (because most berries enjoy being in the sun).

Having settled on a working definition of what a berry is (which is surprisingly difficult in botanical terms, see page 225), we set out to find specimens to use in the recipes: cloudberries in a Scandinavian bog, whortleberries on a remote northern moor, bearberries on a Pyrenean mountainside, jujubes in London's Chinatown, barberries in a local Lebanese shop, sea-buckthorn on a beach, sloes in a hedge, aronia berries near my daughter's school, and others in friends' gardens, farmers' markets, supermarkets and health food stores.

As I searched and researched the subject, I realized that berries are everywhere. They are probably one of the most common foods on the planet, eaten by almost every species as well as by people of every religious and dietary persuasion. And the most amazing thing is that berries are prepared by plants for the *specific* purpose of enticing us to eat them. They come in brilliant colours and bite-size, ready-to-eat packages, bursting with health and requiring no (or very little) cooking. They are easy to dry and freeze, keep all year long and provide perfect protection from disease for migrating birds, people and animals. Writing the berry profiles, I was constantly reminded how incredible it is that such humble and easily accessible foods can have such powerful and universal health benefits: in a world full of food and health hyperbole, berry power really does rule!

Working on the recipes, I discovered that many tribes and indigenous peoples have a long tradition of including berries in all kinds of dishes, from main courses to desserts, as well as the more 'usual' jams, syrups and jellies. Taking their example as my inspiration, I have tried to create a modern take on these old ways and I hope that you, too, will enjoy experimenting with the new tastes and textures that berries can offer.

The joy of finding a perfect, peaceful symbiosis with nature is immense and empowering. To know that I have caused no living being to suffer, or be deprived, by eating my own fair share of berries makes me feel more in tune with my inner self. And since, unlike birds and animals, I tend not to fulfil my part of the bargain by delivering seeds wrapped in fertilizer to new environments, I have instead planted berry bushes in my garden to support their proliferation and provide food for passing wildlife. With urban gardens now sprouting in many parts of the world, I hope that this book will inspire more people to grow berries and to spend more time under open skies, picking this natural source of food and medicine while enjoying the sights, scents and sensations of a simple freedom.

USING THIS BOOK

Botanists use the terms 'fruit' and 'berry' differently from the rest of us. In botanical terms, a berry is a fleshy fruit produced by a plant from a single ovary. Many fruits, such as strawberries, are commonly thought of as berries but do not fit this strict technical definition. On the other hand, bananas, cucumbers, melons and apples are, botanically speaking, berries. So, for practical purposes, it is usual to define berries as small, juicy, edible fruits that are round or oval in shape, sweet to sour in taste, generally brightly coloured and containing seeds or small stones.

In this book, I have decided to include some berries that are normally thought of as vegetables – tomatoes, for example, are probably the most popular berries around the world – and some that are usually considered as fruits (for example, the kiwi fruit and the persimmon). I have also included some small fruits (cherries, damsons and rose hips) that are not berries in the formal botanical sense, but that grow in typical berry habitats, contain similar phytonutrients and are commonly used as food and medicine in the same ways as true berries. Some true berries are not included because, even though they fulfil the technical definition, they are inedible or poisonous, or too easily mistaken for other poisonous fruits or berries.

As you look through the berry profiles and pictures on pages 17–95, you will notice that berries belong to a small number of botanical families and species that share similar characteristics and habitat preferences. Just because *some* berries in a family are edible, however, this does not mean that all berries from that family are safe to eat. For example, goji berries from the *Solanaceae* family are highly nutritious, but the berries of several other plants in the *Solanaceae* group, including the deadly nightshade and the berries of the potato plant are poisonous (although, of course, the potatoes growing underground are safe to eat).

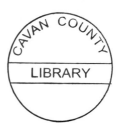

BERRY FACTS

HISTORY, MYTH AND MAGIC

The word 'berry' is at least a thousand years old, though its origin is uncertain. One suggestion is that it comes from the word '*berg*', which in German means mountain, perhaps referring to berries' original, natural environment. Berries are often used as symbols in art and literature, and have multiple cultural, religious and mythological associations. In European folklore, for example, blackberries have been linked with Lucifer and bad omens, and once symbolized sorrow, haste and arrogance. However, they have also been used for protection against malevolent energies and to treat disease. The elderberry was considered mean, and many thought destroying an elder tree would anger the spirit within it causing sorrow and remorse. Yet carrying elderberries about your person was also thought to offer protection from all types of negativity and to bring prosperity.

Raspberries were seen as a symbol of kindness and fragility; strawberries of righteousness and spiritual merit; blueberries of protection; bearberries of psychic powers; and capers of potency, lust and luck. The cherry was for love and divination; and grapes brought fertility, mental powers and prosperity; huckleberry stood for luck, protection and dream magic; and juniper was useful protection during exorcism and against theft. Mulberry and sloes gave protection and strength; Oregon grape attracted money; rowan brought healing, power and success; and cranberries were associated with the abundance of the Earth. And of course, some children are still told that babies come from under a gooseberry bush!

Where this symbolism came from, no one knows, though some of the old beliefs could well be rooted in reason: being well nourished with phytonutrients certainly offers protection, at least from disease, as well as more resources to withstand stress and adversity.

Berry *colour* has also been used as a marker of quality and edibility, although this is clearly unreliable. Red and white berries were often said to be poisonous, for example, but whitecurrants, redcurrants, raspberries, strawberries and rose hips are all extremely delicious and nutritious. Again, it was once thought that all blue and black berries were edible, which is an equally inaccurate belief, as some of the deadly nightshade berries are black. Another myth is that if birds and animals eat a berry then it must be safe for humans too. This is not true, though it does pay to be cautious with any berries that birds do not eat! The berry profiles in this book will help you to identify which ones to leave for the birds, and which ones are the hidden treasures with exquisite flavours and interesting textures to enjoy.

Whatever we may make of the myth and folklore, when it comes to choosing or buying berries to eat it is worth remembering that although big, symmetrical, uniformly coloured, non-juicy berries may have a longer shelf life, they cannot compete for flavour and nutrients with smaller, less even, juicier berries whose *colour* signals their ripeness. Commercially produced berries are bred to be easy to grow, pack, transport and keep on supermarket shelves, and while they can still taste good, they are easily outshone by tiny, wild or locally grown, uneven berries that are picked when ripe and not artificially treated to prolong an appearance of freshness.

ECOLOGY

The berry year begins with the ripening of the first fruits in early summer and continues through the autumn and well into the winter, providing nourishment for wildlife of all kinds. Berries grow on trees, shrubs, climbers and bushes, and provide protection and shelter for many different species, and for the soil itself.

Many of the berries we eat today were present in nature when much of the Earth's land was in its natural state and, although their abundance has been diminished drastically over recent years by forest clearing, intensive farming and urbanization, berry plants continue to grow where no other foods will flourish: from the furthest latitudes to the highest altitudes, and from the driest climates to the poorest soils. Forests, moors, bogs and wastelands, unusable for conventional food growing, provide the perfect habitats for many health-giving berries, and hedgerows and gardens are ideal places for growing and picking nature's own medicines, available to all without prescription or payment.

BERRIES, BIRDS AND ANIMALS

From the plant's perspective, the purpose of producing edible berries is procreation. Most berries have a mutually advantageous relationship with birds and animals in which the plant invests some resources in packaging its precious seeds in a tasty, brightly coloured and nutritious sandwich for wildlife to enjoy. In return, the birds and animals drop the seeds far from the parent plant, usually with a starter kit of natural fertilizer, ready to germinate and establish the species in a new place, hastening the turning of a virtuous natural circle.

Berries come in bite-size portions and are packed with carbohydrates and protein to give the seed carriers the energy and strength to travel far, as well as phytochemicals to keep them healthy en route. Depending on the length of the carrier's digestive system, the seeds are excreted hours – or sometimes days – later. In some cases it seems that plants adapt to become more accessible to particular species, and similarly some birds and animals adapt their anatomy and physiology to become expert berry eaters.

This, at any rate, is how things are supposed to work, but like any win-win situation, the system is vulnerable to cheating: some birds and animals eat berry pulp without spreading the seed, while so-called seed predators, such as parrots, destroy the seed too. Other species are known to eat berries and then dispose of the seeds somewhere inappropriate or inhospitable to berry plants.

BERRIES AND PEOPLE

Hunting for berries is a wonderful pastime. It increases awareness of the natural world around us, and it provides fresh air and exercise that benefits young and old alike. It is fun to find food in hedgerows, backyards and gardens (as most people did until a generation or two ago), and the first bite of a homemade pie containing plump, sun-ripened wild blackberries quickly erases memories of any inconvenience experienced in their picking. Most edible berries have deep, intense, seductive flavours that make them very attractive as natural suppliers of vitamins, minerals and health-promoting phytochemicals, and wild-picked foods are almost certain to be free of sprays and fertilizers, and are inherently organic and GMO-free.

Making the link between our food and the environment it actually comes from is also very empowering, and can become a useful tool in times of need or emergency. Not long ago (and still the case in some parts of the world), knowing where and how to stock up on highly nutritious, immune-boosting berries in preparation for winter was a vital strategy for survival. And knowing just some of the nutritional and medicinal uses for the berries can be useful for promoting and preserving health and wellbeing.

BERRIES FOR HEALTH

Berries are some of the healthiest foods on the planet. For centuries, aboriginal peoples all over the world have relied on them as both food and medicine, and even today people who live close to nature eat an impressive selection of wild berry fruits because of their positive effects on nutrition and health.

The fact that most berries are easy to store and use out of season is an added attraction. Many are easy to dry (including grapes, cranberries and goji berries), and those that are too watery to be dried effectively can be frozen or preserved with alcohol or sugar. The monks of medieval Europe frequently used alcohol to make medicinal tinctures, and many of the liqueurs, wines, syrups and jams that we enjoy today started life as berry-based remedies taken to improve health and overcome disease. Blackcurrants were used as a cough remedy long before they were made into jams and vitamin C drinks, and elderberry wine was once a popular (and effective) treatment for feverish colds.

The American navy once used cranberries to prevent scurvy on long sea voyages in the same way that the British navy once used limes, and many slightly acidic berries have an equally high content of vitamin C, a powerful antioxidant that is important for the maintenance of connective tissues as well as for the healthy function of the immune system. The anthocyanin plant pigments that give some berries their strong blue and red colours are also beneficial to health, acting as antioxidants that can help protect body cells from cancer.

Another berry pigment, lutein, is a carotenoid responsible for a variety of yellow, orange, red and green plant colours. Eating a diet rich in lutein (found in tomatoes and in all yellow, red and orange berries) may help prevent cardiovascular disease and slow the progression of eye disorders such as macular degeneration.

Berries are also popular for the natural sugars they contain and, since many can be eaten raw, they provide a natural, cheap and healthy alternative to confectionery. Encouraging children to substitute some store-bought confectionery with fresh or dried berry fruits can have a significant beneficial impact on their health and wellbeing.

Every month, new research is published describing the health-giving properties of a well-known or recently discovered berry, and there is extensive literature to support the medicinal importance of a wide selection of species. The growing importance of berries as food and medicine reflects their rapidly increasing significance within global fresh produce markets.

In fact, the more that berries are studied, the clearer it becomes that they are the natural powerhouses of the plant kingdom, containing nearly all of the essential amino acids, vitamins, minerals and trace elements necessary for good health. Increasingly, the phytochemicals found in berries are being recognized for their therapeutic and health-giving properties, and the rediscovery by the developed world of berry types known to the indigenous people of many cultures promises exciting pharmacological discoveries in the future. Many foods are tasty, many are good for us, but few can match the simple berry when it comes to promoting health in gentle, delicious ways.

In particular, berries appear to have a significant role to play in the prevention and management of the condition known as metabolic syndrome. As with other medical syndromes, metabolic syndrome refers to a group of associated conditions that act together to raise the risk of serious illness: in this case coronary heart disease, diabetes, strokes and kidney problems. Though there is no single cause, central obesity (fat around the middle), insulin resistance, ageing, hormone changes, lack of exercise and genetic predisposition can all form part of metabolic syndrome, which is becoming increasingly common in industrial and post-industrial societies.

Many different berries have been found to reduce the symptoms related to metabolic syndrome, and eating berries every day is a simple thing that nearly everyone can do to help prevent its development. The underlying mechanism for this effect relates to the proven observation that increased berry consumption (as part of a normal diet) can enhance liver function and reduce levels of tissue inflammation, probably as a result of the high levels of potent antioxidants present in most edible berries. Eating just 150g/5½oz of mixed berries daily has been shown to lower blood cholesterol, reduce the risk of heart disease, stabilize blood sugar and improve insulin resistance.

With such clear health benefits, it is not surprising that berries are becoming big business as scientists extend their research further into making berry-related products to treat a wide range of ailments. The pursuit of profit has fuelled the creation of what some regard as modern myths about berries. For example, açai berries have been hailed as fat burners that will speed up metabolism and promote weight loss; including açai and other berries in your diet – especially at the expense of less nutritious, more fattening foods – will certainly help with the change toward a healthier lifestyle, which in turn helps burn unwanted fat. But the truth is that while açai berries are very nutritious, no single product can give you a flat belly.

Interestingly, it has also been found that the bioactivity of berries depends on the climate and all the environmental conditions that they grow under, which means that eating whole berries is much more beneficial to health than taking medicines made from isolated chemical berry compounds.

In the midst of all the health claims and counterclaims, it is good to remember that the health benefits of berries were here and understood long before we had any scientific evidence, and that berries have always provided a substantial contribution to the health of living beings on this planet. They are easy to grow, require little attention and are easy to store. They are also delicious to eat and to drink, make perfect snacks, tasty packed lunches and convenient foods for journeys; and growing or going out to pick your own is also a healthy, life-enhancing pastime. There really is much to be gained from adopting a berry lifestyle.

EXTENDING THE BERRY SEASON

Although the berry-picking season is short, you can have fresh berries all year by freezing them as soon as they are picked. Choose whole, fully ripe, unblemished berries and freeze them in airtight, resealable bags or boxes, taking care not to squash them. Soft berries, such as raspberries, should be rinsed just before eating, but most berries are easier to strip and rinse before freezing. Ensure that all berries are clean and dry before storing and freezing as excess moisture will hasten decay. Use berries directly from the freezer on breakfast cereals, and for smoothies, desserts and cooked dishes. For cakes and muffins, simply fold frozen berries into the dough just before baking.

THE BERRIES

This chapter will introduce you to the history and habitat, as well as the nutritional, culinary and medicinal properties of 50 common and uncommon berries. Ten berries stand out as 'Super Berries' and are highlighted with pink introductory text (and are in capitals below). You will learn about their wild and wonderful worlds in gardens, hedgerows, wastelands and wildernesses – all natural habitats and places you may pass on your way, perhaps without noticing which berries are tasty and beneficial to eat and which are best avoided. By getting to know which ones are safe, you can find new ways to improve your health and add colour to your diet.

Açai berry	Golden berry	Rose hip
Aronia/Chokeberry	Gooseberry	Rowan
Barberry	GRAPE	Salmonberry
Bearberry	Honeyberry	Sea-buckthorn
Bilberry	Huckleberry	Seagrape
BLACKBERRY	Indian Gooseberry/	Serviceberry
BLACKCURRANT	Amla	Sloe
BLUEBERRY	Jujube/Chinese Date	STRAWBERRY
Boysenberry	Juniper	Strawberry Tree
Caperberry	KIWI FRUIT/CHINESE	Sumac
CHERRY	GOOSEBERRY	Thimbleberry
Cloudberry	Lingonberry	TOMATO
CRANBERRY	Loganberry	Ugniberry
Crowberry	Mulberry	Whitecurrant
Damson	Oregon grape	Whortleberry
Dewberry	Persimmon	Wineberry
ELDERBERRY	Raspberry	
Goji berry	Redcurrant	

Açai berry *Euterpe oleracea*

Açai berries are native to Latin America and grow on large palm trees belonging to the palm tree family (*Arecaceae*). They have long been an important food source for the native Amazonian population, and have recently taken on significant economic value as the health benefits of açai have become more widely appreciated. Although the increased international popularity of the berry has been good for the Brazilian economy, the millions of açai trees planted in the rain forest are posing a problem of 'green deforestation' by turning the old diverse forests into a monoculture of açai palm plantations (though there are increasing numbers of organic plantations with Fairtrade certification). The word 'açai' is a corruption of the Tupian word *ïwaca'i*, meaning 'fruit that expels water', and reflects the fact that the berries have a marked diuretic effect.

The small, round, black-purple açai berry is a drupe, consisting of just 10% pulp and 90% seed. After harvesting, the seeds are removed and the berries are ground to a powder, which is then dried. It takes 8kg/17lb 8oz of fresh berries to produce 1kg/2lb 4oz of açai powder. The pulp and skin can also be made into juice or freeze-dried. Traditionally, the thick, purple fruit pulp is eaten in a porridge/oatmeal combined with fish and manioc, but açai is now found in countless food and health products. The taste is not sweet so it can be used in both savoury and sweet recipes, including ice creams, juices, smoothies, granola bars, liqueurs and sauces. As a health supplement, açai can be bought in tablet, capsule and powder form.

Açai berries help increase energy and stamina, improve immunity, fight infection, control prostate enlargement, support the heart, increase libido, protect against cancer, maintain healthy blood sugar levels, reduce blood cholesterol, ease inflammation and delay the process of ageing. They also suppress appetite, and this ability (in combination with their diuretic action) has made açai berries a popular aid to slimming. Though the claims made for these remarkable berries may sometimes seem exaggerated, their extremely high antioxidant and high protein/low sugar content provides a physiological basis for their beneficial effects on health.

Analysis reveals that 100g/3½oz of powdered açai provides 534 calories, of which 39% is carbohydrate (mainly fibre), 7% is protein and 54% is fat (mainly oleic, palmitic and linoleic acid). It offers vitamins A, B1, B2, B3, C and E, and is rich in minerals, especially potassium and calcium. The pulp has a high fibre content, and contains both omega-9 and omega-6 fatty acids. Eating açai berry pulp regularly over a period of time may lower blood glucose, insulin, cholesterol and LDL levels.

Açai berries may have a higher antioxidant, flavonoid, anthocyanin and phenolic content than red grapes. Anthocyanins give the red to blue colouring to many berries, fruits and vegetables, and are important for a healthy cardiovascular system and to help the immune system deal with malignant cells (there is research evidence that açai berries can destroy leukaemia cells). Phenols are also antioxidants that help to protect body cells from damage caused by free radicals. However, the antioxidant content of açai berries is highly volatile and difficult to store in juice and dried fruits, and it is clear that making açai pulp into juice significantly reduces its health benefits.

Aronia/Chokeberry
Aronia melanocarpa (syn. *Photinia melanocarpa*)

Aronia, or chokeberry, is a woody shrub from the rose family (*Rosaceae*), native to North America. It loves full sun and is often found on the edges of woodland or in hedgerows. The berries grow in end-of-shoot clusters of 10 to 15, and are firm, black and about the same size as blueberries. They ripen in early autumn and can be harvested for several weeks. In strict botanical terms, the aronia berry is a pome, like an apple rather than a berry.

Despite being a year-round decorative garden plant, the aronia berry itself attracts little attention and most people would be unable to identify it. Of those who can, many are unaware of its nutritional and medicinal properties. This is probably because the fresh berries have an extremely dry, astringent taste; even the birds leave them alone during the winter months until all the other berries have been eaten up.

Nevertheless, interest in (and evidence of) the health benefits of the aronia berry has grown markedly in recent years, with commercial production increasing in many parts of the world. It has been cultivated in eastern Europe for many years as a source of vitamin C, and recent research in other parts of the world has established that the antioxidants contained in the berry have huge potential for enhancing human health.

In particular, aronia berries appear to have a role in the prevention and treatment of the major contemporary so-called 'lifestyle diseases', including heart disease and some forms of cancer, as well as chronic inflammation, urinary tract infections and gastrointestinal disorders. Studies investigating the so-called ORAC value (oxygen radical absorbance capacity) of aronia berries show them to have an antioxidant effect on human body cells nearly three times greater than that of blueberries and blackberries, and more than twice as great as the antioxidant effect of blackcurrants and cranberries.

The aronia berry contains significant amounts of vitamins C and E, folate, potassium, magnesium, iron and, particularly, zinc. It is also extremely rich in polyphenol antioxidants, mainly anthocyanins, the pigments responsible for the dark, almost black colour of the berries. Aronia berries are increasingly available fresh or frozen, and also as an ingredient in commercially produced jams, jellies, sauces, ice creams, salsas and, most commonly, fruit juices.

Barberry *Berberis vulgaris*

Barberries are beautiful, flavourful, small, red berries with a taste that resembles cranberries, although they are less bitter than their better-known cousins. They grow on a thorny bush, belonging to the barberry family (*Berberidaceae*), that has very sharp prickles and clusters of yellow flowers, and can be used to make jams and jellies, cakes and wine. Common in Middle Eastern and Asian cuisine, where they are known as *zereshk*, barberries are used to add flavour and colour to rice, couscous and casseroles dishes such as tajines and they taste great with yogurt.

The barberry has a long history as a remedy for digestive ailments, such as poor appetite, heartburn, food poisoning and constipation, and also as an aid to fighting infections including giardiasis, urinary tract infections, colds and influenza. Its anti-inflammatory effect can be helpful in recovery from injury or after intense athletic training, and the high vitamin C content supports the action of the immune system.

Research has shown that barberries are potent against harmful skin bacteria such as *Staphylococcus aureus* and *Streptococcus pyogenes*. These results confirm the traditional use of barberries for skin problems and for soothing sore throats, and reflect the fact that barberries contain significant amounts of an alkaloid called berberine – a strong antimicrobial that inhibits the growth of *E. coli* and other infectious organisms. Several studies have shown that it also has the ability to help the liver clear LDL-cholesterol from the bloodstream and thus reduce the risk of cardiovascular disease.

Barberry tea is made by heating a cupful of water (250ml/8½fl oz) in a pan with 3 teaspoons of whole barberries and simmering for 5–10 minutes before straining. Drinking a cup of barberry tea two to four times a day can be useful to help avoid digestive problems when travelling; start drinking two cups (500ml/17fl oz) per day a week before departure, and take some berries with you to make tea on the way.

WARNING

- Barberries are best avoided if you are pregnant or breast-feeding, or on a medication containing tetracycline. Strong infusions should not be taken for longer than a couple of weeks. Overdosage may cause stomach pain, vomiting, diarrhoea or kidney problems.

Bearberry *Arctostaphylos uva-ursi*

Bearberries, as the name suggests, are part of the staple diet of bears and other North American wildlife, and the Latin name, *uva-ursi*, means bear-grape. Native Americans called them *k'nick* (one of bearberry's common names is kinnikinnick), and used bearberry leaves for smoking as well as adding the berries to flavour cooked dishes, soups and bread.

Bearberries are small, fat and red, and resemble their close relatives, the cranberry and the bilberry. They grow on low bushes, close to the ground, on rocks or on open, dry land, often near pine trees. The plant belongs to the heather family (*Ericaceae*) and is evergreen with small, oblong, leathery leaves and pink, bell-shaped flowers. The berries ripen in late summer and continue appearing until late autumn. They contain a cluster of seeds, and the pulp is dry and mealy when eaten raw, which is why they are also sometimes known as sandberries.

The whole bearberry plant has been used as a medicine in many countries for centuries, especially to treat diarrhoea, dysentery and urinary tract problems, and was first documented by the Physicians of Myddfai in The Red Book of Hergest, a 14th-century collection of Welsh herbal remedies. The bearberry contains arbutin, which is antimicrobial and mildly diuretic, though it is the leaves that contain the highest concentration and are most commonly used to make herbal medicines. The berries can be used as a urinary antiseptic to relieve urinary tract infections, including cystitis (especially when the urine is too acidic), and also as a gentle anti-inflammatory to ease aching joints.

Arbutins are also significant within the cosmetics industry in preparations intended to help inhibit pigment formation, to whiten the skin and remove freckles. A pack of bearberries, steeped in a little water, can be used to soften hard skin, but whether they are able to get rid of freckles is less certain.

Including bearberries in the diet, or making bearberry infusions or syrups, is a gentle way to promote tissue health, externally and internally. Cooking brings out the berries' natural sweetness and, after sieving off the seeds, they make a delicious pale-pink jelly.

Bilberry *Vaccinium myrtillus*

Also known as the European blueberry, this lovely, quite sharp, blue berry is native to the cool heaths, moors, woodlands and mountains of Scandinavia, Europe, Asia, North America and Canada. The way to distinguish a bilberry from the American blueberry is to bite it in half: if it is purple inside, it is a bilberry.

The Latin name *myrtillus* refers to the leaves, which resemble those of the myrtle bush. Bilberries grow paired or singly on a small shrub belonging to the heather family (*Ericaceae*) that prefers damp, sandy, acidic, nutrient-poor soil. They ripen in late summer and have been valued for centuries for their slightly sweet, acidic taste as well as for their nutritional and medicinal qualities. But bilberries are very difficult to grow commercially and do not transport well, so are rarely available in supermarkets, unless frozen. Nowadays they are a popular ingredient in pies, tarts, muffins, jellies and homemade wines.

Records of using bilberries as medicine go back to Hildegard of Bingen (1098–1179), who recommended them to induce menstruation, and they are still used by herbalists to relieve period pain. The dried berries can be used as an infusion to calm diarrhoea, and they have a gentle cooling, astringent, disinfectant effect, which makes them useful in reducing inflammation. They may reduce the incidence of blood clots and atherosclerosis, and their protective effect on collagen helps reduce the ill effects of rheumatoid arthritis and emphysema. Their effect on the microcirculation makes them useful in the management of Raynaud's disease, and they are also used to relieve the symptoms of varicose veins and haemorrhoids.

During the Second World War, it was reported that Royal Air Force pilots used bilberries to improve their night vision during night bombing raids. Since then, studies have shown that eating bilberries can, in fact, influence adjustment to darkness and visual acuity. Further research suggests that bilberries do have the ability to increase blood flow and oxygenation in the eye, making them potentially effective in treating some eye problems including diabetic retinopathy, macular degeneration, cataracts and glaucoma.

Bilberries have a high vitamin C content and also contain tannins, alkaloids, phenolic acids and glucosides, which act synergistically to increase the beneficial effects of bilberries on health. They contain anthocyanins, strong antioxidants that can improve the health of connective tissue, prevent tissue damage by free radicals and suppress histamine release, thus decreasing inflammation. Anthocyanins also decrease capillary fragility and reduce the permeability of the blood-brain barrier. Research shows that bilberries have strong antiviral properties and may be able to inactivate the tick-borne encephalitis (TBE) virus.

BLACKBERRY *Rubus fruticosus, Rubus ulmifolius* and spp

The blackberry is indeed black but it is not actually a berry. It is technically an aggregate fruit consisting of a cluster of small fruits, each called a drupelet, with a seed inside. The best blackberries are ripe for picking from midsummer and the harvest season continues well into the autumn. According to British folklore, blackberries should not be picked after Old Michaelmas Day, 10 October, as the devil was said to claim and spoil them after this date. The warning may have more to do with the fact that the cooler, wetter weather provides the right conditions for the berries to become infected by moulds, making them potentially toxic as well as giving them an unpleasant appearance and flavour.

HABITAT
Blackberries belong to the rose family (*Rosaceae*) and are vigorous perennials that grow in temperate zones all over the world. If you are fortunate enough to live near

a hedgerow, or a wilderness overgrown with brambles, remember that they repay you for the inconvenience of being scratchy, thorny, impassable, invasive weeds by giving the most delicious berries. Bramble means 'prickly', and brambling means enjoying the challenge of picking blackberries, so it is advisable to wear clothes that protect you from being scratched, and that you don't mind getting irreparably stained by the rich, dark anthocyanin pigments in the berries.

Berries growing on the same bramble don't all ripen at the same time. Unripe ones are green, turning pink as they ripen, to glossy black when fully ripe, and fading to a dusty blue-purple when overripe. Only pick the fully ripe ones, as the unripe are unpalatable, acidic and hard, and the overripe ones will disintegrate and stain your fingers and clothes as you try to pick them. Perfect berries come away from the stem easily but are still firm. It is possible, with experience, to know how sweet and ripe a berry is just by the way it feels as you pick it. Firmer berries are best for making jelly, softer ones are perfect in cakes, served with cream, or simply to eat as you pick.

Blackberries are available to buy all over the world, although commercial production of blackberries is concentrated mainly in the United States, Mexico and New Zealand.

PHYTONUTRIENTS
Analysis reveals that 100g/3½oz of blackberries provide 37 calories, and contain 10% protein, 5% fat (no cholesterol), 55% carbohydrate and 29% fibre. They are a very good source of vitamin E (20% RDA), vitamin C (19% RDA), folate (17% RDA), vitamin K, manganese and copper. Blackberries have a high content of antioxidants, especially anthocyanins, and also contain tannins, salicylic acid, ellagic acid, pectin and rutin. The seeds are rich in omega-3 oils that are released when they are chewed.

QUALITIES
The high level of vitamin C makes the blackberry a strong immune booster, helping reduce the risk of colds and infection, as well as some cancers. Blackberry also ranks among the best of antioxidant foods, and recent research has shown blackberry anthocyanins to be effective at inhibiting the growth of colon cancer cells, and at protecting blood vessels against oxidative damage from free radicals.

The cyanidin pigment (which gives blackberries their very dark colour) contains anthocyanin and, together with salicylic acid, this has an anti-inflammatory effect, which can be useful in combating a wide range of diseases, including cancer, arthritis, diabetes and, possibly, Alzheimer's. The ellagic acid content may be helpful in destroying cancer cells and in particular, in reducing the effects of oestrogen metabolism in developing breast cancer cells.

The fibre in blackberries is both soluble and insoluble, and this can help to maintain a healthy digestive system and lower blood cholesterol levels. Taken in moderation, blackberries can be useful in treating simple cases of diarrhoea, but eating too many blackberries can have the opposite effect.

AVAILABILITY AND STORAGE

Pick blackberries in the wild; grow your own; buy them fresh, frozen or dried. Store unblemished fresh berries in the refrigerator for a few days, rinsing just before use, or rinse, dry and freeze (see page 15).

CULINARY USES

Blackberries are delicious in smoothies, juices, jams, desserts, pies, pickles, crumbles, salads, snacks, syrups, cordials and wine.

VARIETIES

The wild blackberry and common blackberry are the best-known varieties, but there are hundreds of other microspecies. The American blackberry and many cultivars are grown commercially. Three types of blackberry bushes are available for growing in gardens: trailing, erect and semi-erect, depending on space and location. Prickle-free cultivars such as 'Loch Ness' and 'Black Diamond' have been developed. The 'Bedford Giant' is a blackberry/raspberry hybrid.

BLACKCURRANT *Ribes nigrum*

Blackcurrants are true berries, produced by a small aromatic shrub belonging to the rose family (*Rosaceae*). The bush has fragrant leaves and stems, and the berries sit in loose clusters of between five and ten. They ripen from glossy green to dark purple in midsummer, with purple flesh containing several seeds.

Early English settlers introduced blackcurrants into North America, where they quickly became popular as both a food and a medicine. But at the beginning of the

20th century, blackcurrants (and other *Ribes* species) were blamed for transferring a fungal disease to pine trees, so the logging industry had them banned from sale. The ban was not lifted until much later in the century, and it is still in place in some states. For this reason, the blackcurrant is not very well known in the United States, although it is making a fast comeback in New York and along some areas on the eastern seaboard, where people have started to appreciate its remarkably high content of health-giving phytonutrients and its wholesome flavour.

During the Second World War, when international trade became disrupted and there was a shortage of oranges in the UK, blackcurrants were recognized as a vital source of vitamin C, so cultivation of the berries was encouraged by the British government. Blackcurrant cordial was distributed free to all children for a number of years from 1942.

Apparently, bears also like eating blackcurrants!

HABITAT

Blackcurrant bushes were once common in the forests of northern Europe and northern Asia, as they prefer cooler climates and tend not to thrive if exposed to too much direct sun. They enjoy slight shade and plenty of mulch and, although they are no longer common in the wild, they are grown commercially all over the cooler parts of the world, notably in New Zealand, Russia, Poland and eastern Europe.

PHYTONUTRIENTS

Analysis reveals that 100g/3½oz of blackcurrants provide 39 calories, and contain 9% protein, less than 1% fat, 68% carbohydrate and 23% fibre. They are a rich source of vitamin C (250% RDA), and also contain significant amounts of vitamins E, B5 and B6, calcium, iron, potassium, copper and manganese. They also contain tannins and anthocyanin pigment, which is responsible for their blue-black-coloured skin.

QUALITIES

Europeans have been growing blackcurrants for food and medicine for 500 years. Blackcurrant juice boiled with sugar was called a *Rob* and considered an excellent remedy for sore throats. Raw juice can also be taken diluted with water to calm fevers. Blackcurrant syrup is useful for relieving coughs and may help to calm whooping cough in children. The very high vitamin C content makes blackcurrants good at helping the immune system deal with common illnesses quickly and efficiently.

The berries have a unique, tart flavour, partly because of their high vitamin C content. They can help protect against cardiovascular problems, cancer and a wide range of infections, and their potassium content makes them useful diuretics, which can be helpful in the treatment of high blood pressure and diabetes. They have also shown potential to fight heart disease, infections and neurological disorders.

Blackcurrant seeds contain vitamin E, GLA (gamma-linolenic acid) and omega oils, which help to improve the effectiveness of the immune system and are also used for treating hormonal problems, painful periods and breast tenderness. Applied directly to the skin, GLA and omega oils can be used to relieve dermatitis.

These powerful antioxidant berries can also be used to reduce inflammation and support the management of arthritis, gout and liver problems as well as aid the treatment of capillary fragility, high blood pressure, kidney stones and colic.

AVAILABILITY AND STORAGE

Grow your own blackcurrants; buy them fresh, frozen or dried, or in drinks. Store fresh blackcurrants in the refrigerator for a few days. Rinse just before use, or rinse, dry and freeze (see page 15).

CULINARY USES

Delicious raw in smoothies, juices and salads, blackcurrants are a popular ingredient in cordials and in the French liqueur Crème de Cassis (see page 221). They are also excellent cooked in pies, cakes, confectionery, jams, jellies and preserves.

VARIETIES

There is an increasing range of blackcurrant varieties available as nurserymen are developing new cultivars all the time, trying to improve the quality of the fruit, the productivity of the plants, and to make the bushes stronger and more resistant to frost and diseases. Research continues in North America to produce varieties that are resistant to white pine blister rust (the fungal disease that led to blackcurrants being banned), while also producing a good yield of easily cropped fruit. The current most popular variety for growing in gardens is 'Ben Hope', along with other cultivars 'Ben Lomond' and 'Ben Connan'.

A new green blackcurrant with a sweeter, milder flavour has been cultivated in Finland. Further research into breeding new varieties continues in New Zealand, Sweden, Russia, Poland, Scotland and North America.

BLUEBERRY *Vaccinium cyanococcus*

The blueberry is dark blue, about 1cm/½in across with a flared crown at the end. It is pale green at first, changing to red and then purple before turning deep blue when ripe. Blueberries have a distinctive sweet, slightly acidic taste and their popularity means they are grown commercially all over the globe, making it possible to enjoy them fresh almost all year round.

HABITAT

Blueberries belong to the heather family (*Ericaceae*) and grow wild throughout North America, Europe and Asia, and are often mistaken for another blue berry, the bilberry (see pages 22–23), which is also commonly gathered and eaten in Europe. It is easy to distinguish between the two by cutting the berries in half: ripe blueberries have white or greenish flesh, while bilberries are coloured purple throughout.

The leaves can be either deciduous or evergreen, with or without finely toothed edges. The flowers are bell-shaped, white, pale pink or red and appear from late spring into summer, while the berries ripen at different times from early summer into autumn.

These days, blueberry plants come in several varieties: 'lowbush blueberries' are wild, 10–30cm/4–12in high shrubs, while the 'highbush' variety (which is grown commercially) can reach up to 4m/13ft high. New cultivars are easy to grow in the garden, preferring a slightly acidic habitat in good compost, and there is a certain satisfaction in having a visitor from the wild residing in a corner of the garden, bringing tasty gifts to all its inhabitants.

PHYTONUTRIENTS

Analysis reveals that 100g/3½oz of blueberries provide 59 calories, and contain 5% protein, 5% fat, 82% carbohydrate and 8% fibre. They also contain vitamins A,C, E, K, B1, B2, B3 and B6, folate, potassium, manganese, copper, antioxidants (anthocyanins and flavonoids), mucilage and tannins.

QUALITIES

Blueberries make tasty, low-calorie snacks and can be enjoyed fresh, dried or frozen. They are an ideal natural dietary supplement as they are packed with nutrients while being low in sugars and fat.

In health terms, the blueberry deserves its reputation as the antioxidant superberry because its high levels of powerful antioxidants and tannins help to protect body cells by neutralizing free radicals in the bloodstream, thus reducing the risk of cancer and degenerative illnesses. In recent research into more than 20 different fruits and berries, blueberries were found to have the highest antioxidant capacity and were shown to be capable of inhibiting cancer cell development, dampening inflammation and reducing the likelihood of contracting viral and other infections.

Eating blueberries on a regular basis has been found to increase memory and learning ability and can lessen symptoms of depression – so they may be useful in the management of Alzheimer's disease. Also, blueberries offer cardiovascular benefits as they can lower the levels of blood cholesterol, and so may help to prevent heart disease and high blood pressure. Their toning effect on blood vessels is also useful in the treatment of varicose veins and haemorrhoids.

The tonic and antibacterial properties of blueberries are most marked in the dried berries, which can be used as a simple and effective treatment for diarrhoea. Like cranberries, their close relative, blueberries also contain a mucilage that protects the lining on the urinary tract and prevents bacteria from attaching themselves to the bladder wall, so blueberries can be beneficial in the management of cystitis and other urinary tract infections. The anthocyanin content of blueberries may also improve night vision and eyesight, as well as ease tired eyes.

People with diabetes can also benefit from the blueberry's low glycaemic index as well as its potential to lower blood sugar. Dieters can enjoy them as a low-calorie, low-fat, high-fibre supplement to their regime as they are also thought to help burn fat and increase metabolic health. In recent years, they have become increasingly popular for their therapeutic effects as well as for their great taste – the blueberry muffin being unsurpassed in popularity among cake-lovers of all ages.

AVAILABILITY AND STORAGE
Pick blueberries in the wild; grow your own; buy fresh, frozen or dried, or in drinks. Store unblemished fresh berries in the refrigerator for a week or so. Rinse just before use, or freeze (see page 15).

CULINARY USES
Blueberries are delicious baked in muffins and pies; made into jams and jellies, juices, smoothies and wine; or sprinkled on breakfast cereals, salads and desserts.

VARIETIES

Many different varieties of blueberry are grown around the world. Some of the best known are: Alaska blueberry (*Vaccinium alaskaense*), lowbush blueberry (*V. angustifolium*), northern blueberry (*V. boreale*), New Jersey blueberry (*V. caesariense*), highbush blueberry (*V. corymbosum*), American blueberry (*V. cyanococcus*), southern blueberry (*V. formosum*), evergreen blueberry (*V. myrsinites*), black highbush blueberry (*V. fuscatum*), hairy-fruited blueberry (*V. hirsutum*), Canadian blueberry (*V. myrtilloides*), cyan-fruited blueberry (*V. operium*), dryland blueberry (*V. pallidum*) and rabbit-eye blueberry (*V. virgatum*).

Boysenberry *Rubus ursinus x idaeus*

A cross between a raspberry, a blackberry and a loganberry, the boysenberry belongs to the rose family (*Rosaceae*) and was first developed and grown on a farm in California in the 1920s by a farmer named Rudolph Boysen. However, before Boysen was able to establish his berry as a commercial crop, he broke his back in an accident and abandoned the farm.

It was not until some years later that a fellow berry grower, Walter Knott, tracked him down and managed to nurture some of the dying vines back to health, and so it was Knott's berry farm (also in California) that established the boysenberry as a popular fruit. Boysenberries are now available almost everywhere: frozen, puréed, as a concentrate, as well as in a variety of foods and drinks, including jams, yogurts and preserves. Unfortunately, fresh berries are not easy to buy as they are soft and difficult to handle without bruising, making them almost impossible to transport undamaged.

In botanical terms, the boysenberry is classified as a compound fruit that presents a large seed in each segment. The canes are easy to grow and the berries are easy to pick if they are trained up a wall or fence with wire frames or trellises. They are delicate plants that prefer a mild climate and need mulching in winter to protect them from frost. With their rich, deep reddish-purple colour and sweet, intense flavour, boysenberries have grown increasingly popular as a food, which has led to increased interest in studying their health benefits. They are high in folate, ellagic acid, vitamin K and manganese, and also in antioxidants, anthocyanins, ellagitannins, gallic acid and dietary fibre, making them helpful in reducing high blood cholesterol (which in turn reduces the risk of cardiovascular disease).

Boysenberries also have anti-inflammatory and wound-healing properties, and there is evidence that they can help prevent breast cancer. Ellagic acid has been found to reduce the effect of oestrogen on hormone-sensitive cancer cells, and helps the liver to rid the blood of circulating carcinogens. Gallic acid is thought to inhibit adenocarcinomas, reducing the growth of prostate cancer cells and malignant tumours in other glands. A recent study also showed that the anthocyanins in boysenberries are effective at reducing the effects of free radicals, which are thought to play a role in neurodegenerative diseases such as MS, ME, Parkinson's and Alzheimer's disease.

Caperberry *Capparis spinosa*

Caperberries come from the caper bush, also known as 'Flinders rose', belonging to the caper family (*Capparaceae*), which grows throughout the Mediterranean and other regions that have hot, dry, sunny climates, such as California. The origin of the caper plant is unknown, but it is thought to have developed in Asia. Capers and caperberries are not the same thing: capers are the edible flower buds of the bush, while the caperberry is a true berry that develops from the flower.

The berries have a distinctive, aromatic flavour that develops when they are pickled in vinegar, brine or salt. They are the size of an olive, have faint white stripes and sit on a long stalk. Delicious as a snack or a condiment, they are used traditionally to add a piquant pungency to Mediterranean dishes, pasta sauces, pizzas and salads.

Caperberries were used in ancient Greek and Roman times to promote digestion and relieve wind, and were also thought to have aphrodisiac properties. Pickling causes the release of mustard oil and large amounts of the antioxidant bioflavonoids rutin and quercetin. Rutin is known to strengthen capillary walls and inhibit platelet aggregation, thus helping circulation in small blood vessels. Quercetin is antibacterial, anti-carcinogenic and anti-inflammatory.

Caperberries are low in calories but high in protein (32%), fibre (21%), omega-3 and omega-6 oils, vitamins E and B2, iron and copper. The high plant-protein content slows the absorption of carbohydrates and helps prevent sudden blood sugar rises. It can also help prevent overeating, as protein stimulates the brain's hunger control centres.

Caperberries have been found to reduce the negative impact of eating saturated fats and red meat by helping to prevent the formation of digested by-products linked to an increased risk of cancer and heart disease. Research also shows that caperberries can help prevent the oxidation of fat during cooking (and during digestion), and that they can help maintain vitamin E levels in the body. Herbalists also use caperberries for the treatment of haemorrhoids and varicose veins.

CHERRY *Prunus avium* and *Prunus cerasus*

Although shaped like a berry, a cherry contains just a single stone, so by botanical definition it is really a drupe belonging to the rose family (*Rosaceae*). Cherries ripen in the early summer and are among the first fresh berries of the season. Fresh, locally grown cherries are available for only a very short season because they ripen almost simultaneously on the tree, but as they are grown commercially in both the Northern and Southern Hemispheres, they are always in season somewhere in the world.

Since 1915, Traverse City in the American state of Michigan has hosted an annual National Cherry Festival where the inhabitants enjoy pit-spitting competitions, pie-eating contests, attempts to make the world's biggest cherry pie and the crowning of the Cherry Queen. According to its citizens, Traverse is 'The Cherry Capital of the World'.

HABITAT

A cherry seed needs exposure to cold in order to germinate. Consequently, cherry trees grow only in temperate climates and are not found in the tropics. They take three to four years to produce their first crop of berries and seven years to reach maturity. The more sun these trees receive in a season, the sweeter their cherries will taste, and as they prefer cool winters and hot sun, cherry trees are well suited to growing in mountain areas.

Cherries are grown commercially in the sunniest regions of Europe, Scandinavia, the Baltic States, the southern parts of Australia and in most of North America. Turkey, the United States, Iran, Italy and Spain are the world's main producers. More than two million tonnes of cherries are grown commercially each year, with perhaps another million growing on trees in private gardens and in the wild.

PHYTONUTRIENTS

Analysis reveals that 100g/3½oz of cherries provide 48 calories, and contain 7% protein, 3% fat, 82% carbohydrate and 8% fibre. They also contain vitamins C (14% RDA), B1, B5 and B6, folate, potassium and magnesium. They have a high melatonin content and are packed with antioxidants, especially anthocyanin, melanin, flavonoids (lutein, zeaxanthin, carotenoids), phenols and quercetin.

QUALITIES

The anthocyanins in cherries have been shown to be powerful anti-inflammatory agents, capable of reducing pain and swelling from gout, arthritis, fibromyalgia and injuries. They can also help the body to fight cancer, neurological problems, cell deterioration and diabetes. Flavonoids act as protective scavengers against free radicals, reducing the risk of heart disease, cancer and other chronic disease processes.

Eating cherries or drinking cherry juice can help to improve your natural sleep cycle. It can also be a good remedy for insomnia as melatonin, a natural hormone produced by plants, animals and people, plays a key role in regulating the internal body clock. In addition, melatonin helps maintain optimum brainpower and may slow the development of age-related chronic diseases, such as Alzheimer's. The combination of melatonin and anthocyanins makes cherries an excellent brain food.

Cherries are good to eat as a snack when dieting or on a weight control regime, and can help to reduce joint pain and inflammation after vigorous exercise.

AVAILABILITY AND STORAGE

Pick cherries in the wild; grow your own; or buy them fresh, dried, tinned, pickled or frozen, or in food products or drinks. Bright, shiny cherries with green stalks firmly attached can be refrigerated for about a week. Rinse just before eating, or you can freeze rinsed and dried whole cherries for up to a year.

CULINARY USES

Cherries make excellent snacks and are good in salads, drinks, juices, syrups, cakes, ice cream, chocolates and desserts.

VARIETIES

There are countless species of cherries, but the two most popular types are the sweet cherry (*Prunus avium*) and the sour cherry (*P. cerasus*). Other varieties include

Alabama cherry (*P. alabamensis*), clove cherry (*P. apetala*), bell-flowered cherry
(*P. campanulata*), greyleaf cherry (*P. canescens*), Carolina cherry laurel (*P. caroliniana*),
wild Himalayan cherry (*P. cerasoides*), Oregon cherry or bitter cherry (*P. emarginata*),
European/Asian bird cherry (*P. padus*), black cherry (*P. serotina*), Tibetan cherry
(*P. serrula*), Hokkaido bird cherry (*P. ssiori*), Korean mountain cherry (*P. verecunda*),
chokecherry (*P. virginiana*) and Yoshino cherry (*P. x yedoensis*).

Cloudberry *Rubus chamaemorus*

There is a consensus among climate scientists that global warming is happening
much faster in the Arctic regions and alpine areas than anywhere else in the
world, and that the changes are already affecting the vegetation. Many Arctic
and alpine plants thrive because there is little or no competition from other
species. With increasing average seasonal temperatures, more plants start to
compete for resources with the existing flora.

Cloudberries inhabit peaty moors and bogs, mainly in cool, remote, mountainous
areas where the soil is acidic and poor in nutrients, and this elusive shrub is one of
the plants under threat. The cloudberry is slowly losing its habitat, and temperature
stress is affecting its metabolism and the nutrients and phytochemicals it produces.

Also known as dwarf mulberry and bakeapple to Nordic people, the orange-
to amber-coloured cloudberry is described by some as 'the queen of Scandinavian
berries'. It is capricious and unpredictable – some years bountiful, others hardly
present – and in years of plenty, the ground is covered in golden berries spreading
a magical light up from the earth.

Technically classified as composite fruits rather than berries, cloudberries
belong to the rose family (*Rosaceae*). They are truly delicious with a sweet aromatic
juice and have always been part of the Scandinavian diet. They can be eaten fresh
or frozen, in ice creams, jams, jellies, pies, wines, liqueurs, desserts and syrups.
Though primarily a wild plant, cloudberry is now produced commercially in northern
Scandinavia and Arctic areas where few other crops will grow (a task made easier
by the fact that they keep well, making them relatively easy to store and transport).

The cloudberry has a remarkably high vitamin C content, with 100g/3½oz
providing more than two and a half times the recommended daily allowance.

It is also rich in iron, copper, zinc, potassium, calcium and magnesium, as well as important phytochemicals such as salicylic acid, benzoin, quercetin, kaempferol, carotenoids, ellagitannins and leucoanthocyanins. The seeds are rich in vitamin E and phytosterols as well as omega fatty acids similar to those found in evening primrose. These nutrients have many biological properties beneficial to human health including the inhibition of genetic mutations that may lead to the development of cancer cells. They also help support liver function and strengthen the immune system's ability to fight infectious disease. Externally, cloudberry preparations can be used to treat burns and skin infections, and to encourage wound healing.

CRANBERRY *Vaccinium oxycoccos, Vaccinium macrocarpon* and *Vaccinium erythrocarpum*

The cranberry is a small, round, true berry, about 8mm/⅜in in diameter. It grows on thin, thread-like stems, and is initially white but turns deep red, with a characteristic sweet-acidic, tangy taste when fully ripe. There are several theories concerning the origin of the name 'cranberry'. One is that the open flowers resemble the head and bill of a crane; another is that cranes like eating them. Native Americans called the berry *ibimi*, meaning 'bitter berry', and used it as a food, a medicine and a symbol of peace. Nowadays, cranberries are a major commercial crop in the United States and Canada. In 1996, the worldwide cranberry harvest was reported to produce at least 40 cranberries for every person on the planet. Today, most of the cranberries grown commercially are processed into juice drinks and preserves or condiments.

HABITAT
Cranberries belong to the heather family (*Ericaceae*) and grow in acidic peat bogs in the cooler regions of the Northern Hemisphere. Low-growing shrubs or creeping vines with small evergreen leaves and dainty pink flowers, they appear in early summer, although the berries do not ripen until the autumn. Cranberries and lingonberries (see pages 54–55) are very similar in appearance, but the cranberry thrives on very little fertilizer, while the lingonberry is more greedy. The result is that wild cranberries have disappeared and lingonberries now thrive in areas where intensive farming is the norm and excess fertilizer runs off into the surrounding lands and waterways.

PHYTONUTRIENTS

Analysis reveals that 100g/3½oz of cranberries provide 23 calories, and contain 7% protein, 4% fat, 56% carbohydrate and 33% fibre. They also provide vitamins C (16% RDA), B1, B5, B6, E and K, iron, copper and manganese, and are rich in tannins, antioxidants, salicylic acid, flavonoids and phenols.

QUALITIES

Cranberries are not only sour but also very bitter to taste, being almost impossible to eat on their own. Yet adding a little bit of sweetness from other berries or fruits reveals a whole new quality and dishes can take on a new intensity of flavour when cranberries are added.

These little crimson berries have received much attention from the medical world for a long time because of their usefulness against both chronic and acute urinary tract infections. Research suggests that they can be more effective than common antibiotics in the management of acute cystitis, since the proanthocyanidins in cranberries help to reduce the ability of bacteria to stick to the walls of the urinary tract. Other research has shown that men with prostate problems, who were treated with cranberries for urinary tract infections, also noticed a marked improvement to any other symptoms that had been caused by chronic prostatitis or an enlarged prostate gland.

Cranberries contain significant amounts of important antioxidants that can benefit the heart and circulation, increase immunity and help prevent cancer. Their polyphenol content gives them the ability to limit inflammation and enhances their antibiotic and antioxidant effects. They have also been shown to inhibit the growth of *Helicobacter pylori*, the bacteria that is responsible for causing some types of stomach ulcers.

If you chew a fresh cranberry, the tannins in the juice contract the tissues in the gums and block the pathogens that cause tooth decay, so cranberry can be used to prevent and treat dental plaque and gingivitis.

Even before the discovery of vitamin C, 19th-century American and Canadian sailors on long voyages knew that eating cranberries could protect them from scurvy. The berries were kept fresh in barrels of water and their reputation as a natural vitamin C supplement continues to this day.

WARNING

- If you take the blood-thinning medicine warfarin, you should check whether you are genetically predisposed to increased sensitivity to this drug before drinking cranberry juice.

AVAILABILITY AND STORAGE

Pick wild cranberries; grow your own or buy fresh, frozen or dried, or in food products and drinks. Fresh cranberries can be stored in a refrigerator for up to one month or in a freezer for up to nine months. Do not wash them until just before use.

CULINARY USES

Cranberries are best when juiced or pickled; in sauces, wine and jelly; or cooked in soups, savoury dishes, desserts, scones/soda biscuits and cakes.

VARIETIES

Cranberries used to be picked in the wild and had names that described their characteristics, such as 'Early Black' or 'Early Red'. Later varieties were named after the people who grew them, including 'Howes' and 'McFarlin', or after the place they came from, for example, 'Beavers' from Nova Scotia or 'Jerseys' from New Jersey.

Nowadays, there are more than 100 different cultivars including 'Aviator', 'Bugle', 'Black Veil' or 'Metallic Bell', 'Ben Lears', 'Pilgrims', 'Stevens', 'Bergmans', 'Middleboro', 'Middlesex' or 'Rhode Island'. These newer varieties produce larger berries than the originals.

Crowberry *Empetrum nigrum*

Crowberries are small black drupes (having a stone in the middle), that resemble blueberries but are smaller and darker. They grow on a dwarf evergreen shrub belonging to the heather family (*Ericaceae*), which prefers cool to cold climate conditions and sandy soil, and can be found on moorlands, tundra, sand dunes and in pine forests. Like cloudberries, they have played an important role in the native diets and medicines of the people of the Nordic countries and Arctic regions.

Crowberries can be picked from the middle of summer until the first snows arrive, although their flavour is considered best at the start of the season. However, as they are easy to store, crowberries used to be harvested traditionally in the autumn and kept as part of the winter food supply. They give a steady harvest year after year, and keep well on the bush until the following spring.

Although crowberries are described as being watery, quite tart and bitter when eaten raw, cooking improves their flavour and they can be enjoyed in pies and jellies, wine, desserts and ice creams. They can also be used raw in juices, berry soups and porridge/oatmeal, as well as to add colour and flavour to stews and casseroles.

Crowberries have a high water content and are low in calories. They are high in fibre and protein (27%), and rich in vitamins C, E, K and B-complex (especially pantothenic acid, the 'anti-stress' vitamin). They also contain significant amounts of copper and manganese, and phytochemicals including tannins and antioxidant anthocyanins.

In traditional medicine, crowberries have been used for treating epilepsy, paralysis and nervous disorders, and their high anthocyanin content makes them useful in the management of degenerative diseases. They are diuretic and can reduce blood pressure and the fragility and permeability of the small blood vessels, and so help to strengthen the heart and circulation.

The tannins in crowberries have an astringent effect that can be useful in the treatment of some gastrointestinal conditions and skin problems. They act on proteins to bind the tissues together and form a protective layer on mucous membranes and thus can be useful in the treatment of diarrhoea, bleeding, inflammation or infection.

Damson *Prunus insititia*

Sometimes called wild plum or damask plum, the name 'damson' comes from its original Latin name, *Prunum damascenum*, which translates as 'plum of Damascus', where it is believed the fruit was first cultivated. The Romans brought damsons to England and, many generations later, English settlers introduced them to North America.

The damson is an oval drupe with yellow-green flesh and dark indigo skin. It grows on a small tree belonging to the rose family (*Rosaceae*) that flowers in spring and starts to ripen at the end of summer. Damson skin is tart and the flesh is juicy yet acidic, so raw damsons are not to everyone's taste. However, when cooked, damsons make fine jams and jellies, and are tasty in pies and sauces. They are also used to make wines, damson gin (which is made in the same way as sloe gin), and the famous Slavic *Slivovitz* damson brandy (see page 223).

Traditionally, damsons were used as a remedy for constipation. They are low in calories and high in fibre, vitamins A, C, K and B6, and potassium. Vitamin C encourages efficient absorption of iron from the diet and, together with vitamin A, helps protect against age-related macular degeneration (ARMD), the primary cause of loss of vision in older adults. Vitamins C and K also act to boost the immune system, protect against infection, lower blood pressure and reduce blood fat and cholesterol levels.

As well as vitamins and minerals, damsons contain carotenoids, pectin, chlorogenic, malic and tartaric acids, flavonoids, including anthocyanins, and other antioxidants. Recent understanding of the importance of antioxidants in the diet has revealed many of the health benefits that are gained from these small natural food supplements. The antioxidants in damsons have a high ORAC value (oxygen radical absorbance capacity), which can help the body deal with the free radicals that are associated with the degenerative changes that come with ageing.

Dewberry *Rubus caesius*

In temperate parts of the Northern Hemisphere, dewberries are common weeds that thrive in poor, well-drained soils and act as pioneer plants at the edges of forests and clearings, waysides and hedgerows, grasslands and sand dunes. The berries resemble early blackberries but are smaller and look more like a deep purple or black raspberry covered with a thin layer of waxy, dew-like droplets. The plants bloom in spring, then the white flowers turn into small green berries that change colour and ripen in the middle of summer. Dewberry plants belong to the rose family (*Rosaceae*) and grow on the ground like vines, and the stems are covered with fine spikes that make picking dewberries a scratchy job.

Dewberry leaves can be used to make a pleasant tisane and the berries are aromatic and juicy, if a little tart. They are delicious eaten raw and cooked in juices, jams, jellies, crumbles and pies.

Interest in the dewberry's phytochemical content has led to an increase in their commercial production, and the fact that they are so easy to grow (tolerating both hot and cold weather, as well as drought) has enhanced their popularity. Dewberries are astringent, anti-inflammatory and immune boosting, and can be used to calm fevers, relieve diarrhoea and other gastrointestinal problems, and even to treat worms. They are low in calories (59 per 100g/3½oz) and fat, and relatively high in protein and fibre. They are also rich in vitamins E, C, thiamin, riboflavin and folate, and contain a variety of antioxidants that help protect body cells from oxidation damage.

ELDERBERRY AND BLUE ELDERBERRY *Sambucus nigra* and *Sambucus caerulea*

The elderberry tree used to belong to the honeysuckle family (*Caprifoliaceae*) but has recently been included in the mochatel family (*Adoxaceae*). It is easy to recognize in the summer with its cheerful clusters of white flowers and its aromatic, slightly acidic scent. As autumn approaches, the flowers turn into beautiful green, true berries that change colour as they ripen, becoming white, then red and finally, indigo-black. The ripe berries are very popular among wild birds and animals, and in Scandinavia they are bottled and used to make cordials and elderberry soup.

Known to Native Americans as 'The Tree of Music', the elder was often used to make whistles and flutes because of its straight, woody, pith-centred branches. These properties also made it popular in the production of makeshift snorkels, pipes, blowguns and pea-shooters (would-be whittlers should take note that the sap of the leaves, the wood and the roots all contain poisonous cyanogenic glycosides that can cause allergic and toxic reactions).

The Romans used elderberry juice as a hair dye, a practice that continued into the Middle Ages with renowned herbalist Nicholas Culpeper writing that 'the hair of the head washed with the berries boiled in wine is made black'. The berries were also held in high esteem for their efficacy against rheumatic complaints and skin infections. Elderberry juice was used to treat arthritis and syphilis, and as a laxative, since it was thought 'to promote all fluid secretions and natural evacuations...'.

HABITAT

Elderberries can be found in open woods, along roadsides and in hedgerows, and usually grow in clumps of small, upright, round stems up to 3m/10ft tall. They bloom from late spring to midsummer, displaying distinctive, flat-topped or domed umbels of creamy-white flowers that turn into abundant clusters of tiny, round, green berries that ripen to blue-black in the autumn.

PHYTONUTRIENTS

Analysis reveals that 100g/3½oz of elderberries provide 47 calories, and contain 6% protein, 9% fat, 57% carbohydrate and 28% fibre. They are rich in vitamin C (34% RDA), vitamin A (8% RDA) and iron (11% RDA), and also contain vitamins B1, B2, B3, B5 and B6, folate, biotin, potassium and calcium, together with flavonoids, anthocyanins, rutin, quercetin, viburnic acid, tannins and glycosides.

QUALITIES

Once a staple ingredient in many North American and European dishes, elderberries have been overlooked in recent years as people have moved away from growing and gathering food for themselves.

Elderberries contain potent, antiviral phytochemicals, which can relieve the symptoms of colds and influenza. They are also thought to be effective against herpes and other immune deficiency disorders. Recent studies suggest that the flavonoids in elderberries may be more effective than Tamiflu in treating the symptoms of flu viruses.

AVAILABILITY AND STORAGE

As fresh elderberries do not keep well, they are rarely found for sale in shops or markets. Pick them in the wild or grow your own. The berries are ripe when the clusters start to point downward. Cut or break off whole stalks and rinse well. It's easier to strip the berries from their stems once they are frozen, so freeze elderberries at this stage if you wish. Dry them off well before placing in the freezer in an airtight bag or container, taking care not to squash them. De-stem them while they are frozen by pushing them off with a fork. Occasionally you can buy elderberries frozen or dried, or in food products and drinks.

CULINARY USES

Nibble raw, ripe elderberries directly from the tree, or use them in pancakes, waffles, pies, muffins, sauces, soups, salads, juices and smoothies. The fresh berries can taste slightly bitter, but this can be countered by adding a little lemon juice or some sour apples. They can also be dried or preserved in wine, syrup, cordial, jelly and jam.

VARIETIES

There are at least 30 species of shrubs and small trees called 'Elder' that are commonly grown around the world, but the name is usually taken to refer to the black elder, which is found throughout Europe and North America. Regional subspecies include: American elder; southern elder; Chinese elder; Madeira elder; Canary Island elder; Peruvian elder; Florida elder and Velvet elder.

Goji berry *Lycium barbarum*

Goji berries, also known as wolfberries, have been used in Asia as food and medicine since 2800 BC, and traditionally they were used to increase longevity and to treat poor eyesight, kidney disease and liver disorders. They are still used in traditional Chinese and Japanese medicine for many conditions relating to the eye, and also for hormonal imbalances, fatigue, dizziness and urinary tract problems. Interest in the medicinal properties of goji berries has spread around the world in recent years and this attention has given rise to a stream of goji-based commercial health products. Goji sales are now big business – Chinese exports alone generated US$120 million in 2004 – and recent research suggests that these small red berries may indeed be effective in the management of sexual dysfunction, glaucoma, diabetes and various other, mainly age-related, health problems.

The goji plant belongs to the nightshade family (*Solanaceae*) and is a deciduous woody perennial climber, growing up to 3m/10ft high. Bell-shaped flowers appear during the summer and are lavender or light purple in colour. The elongated berries are bright crimson when they ripen in late summer or early autumn, and are about 1–2cm/½–¾in long. Gojis are true berries in the botanical sense, each containing between 10 and 60 tiny yellow seeds. Ripe gojis are difficult to harvest as they bruise easily, so it is best to shake them gently into trays and dry them slowly, out of direct sunlight, with minimum handling.

As a food, goji berries can be eaten dried, juiced or extracted in alcohol. Dried goji berries taste like a combination of raisins and cranberries and are a tasty and healthy addition to any meal. They are high in protein (36%) and fibre, and in vitamins C and B1, as well as calcium and iron.

Research into the health effects of goji berries has concentrated mainly on their *L.barbarum* polysaccharide (LBP) content. LBP has been shown to help reduce body weight, and clinical trials on diabetics have suggested that it also improves circulation and immunity. Goji berries contain carotenoids, including lutein, which may prevent oxidative damage to the retina of the eye, and they also contain flavonoids, phenolic acids and other powerful antioxidants.

Eating goji berries stimulates the immune system, lessens inflammation and can speed up recovery after chemotherapy or radiation. Studies involving cancer patients have shown inhibited growth or regression of cancer cells, and goji berries have also been shown to alter oestradiol metabolism, and may thus affect female hormonal cancers in a positive way. Other clinical studies suggest that eating goji berries increases energy levels, stamina and endurance; improves sleep quality and mental alertness; and reduces the incidence of headache, depression and memory loss.

Golden berry *Physalis peruviana*

Also known as cape gooseberry, groundcherry, inca berry and *poha*, this tasty berry is native to the tropical mountains of South America where it still grows wild. Over the centuries, the golden berry has been introduced to most parts of the world by travellers enthusiastic about its juicy, sweet and slightly acidic gooseberry-like flavour; its plentiful nutrients; and its ability to keep fresh for weeks without special treatment. In the 18th century it was grown in South Africa by early settlers at the Cape of Good Hope, hence the name 'cape gooseberry'.

The golden berry is easy to recognize: a small, round, bright yellow berry sitting inside its own papery pod resembling a Chinese lantern. A true berry containing numerous little yellow seeds, it belongs to the nightshade (*Solanaceae*) family and is closely related to the Mexican tomatillo. The golden berry plant is a small perennial bush that grows up to about 1m/3ft high and flowers from the middle of summer to the middle of autumn, with the berries ripening from the end of summer to the end of autumn. It prefers well-drained, moist soil and can grow in semi-shade or full sun, but it needs frost protection in winter.

Eaten fresh in snacks and salads, golden berries are a common ingredient in jams, muffins, pies, crumbles, sorbets and other desserts. The berries can also be dried or sun-dried, and in the process they take on a lovely, complex, sweet and sour, citrus-like flavour. In recent years the golden berry has become a commercially important crop in many parts of the world.

The golden berry has long been used in traditional medicine as an aid to slimming and weight control, and also to boost immunity, lower cholesterol, reduce the frequency and severity of asthma attacks and dampen allergic reactions. Modern research seems to confirm these uses, and also suggests that eating golden berries may help to inhibit the growth of cancer cells. The health-promoting phytochemicals underlying these properties include flavonoids (vitamin P), polyphenols, phytosterols, physalin glycosides and carotenoids.

A low-calorie, high-protein, high-fibre food, golden berries contain omega oils and essential fatty acids; vitamins A, C, E, K, thiamin and niacin; and minerals phosphorus, potassium, zinc and iron.

Gooseberry *Ribes uva-crispa* (syn. *R. grossularia*)

Native to Europe, North Africa and south Asia, gooseberries are an ancient species first mentioned in English records in 1276. By the middle of the 1700s nearly every garden in Britain featured a plant and the gooseberry had become so popular that gooseberry clubs were formed with members competing to produce the biggest and best specimens, some as large as kiwi fruit. The fruit fell out of favour in the latter part of the 20th century, but a few clubs still exist today and people's taste for gooseberries seems to have been rekindled.

In the 1920s, the US government banned the production and sale of gooseberries as one of the *Ribes* species, believing them to be partly responsible for a fungal disease affecting pine trees that was damaging the timber industry. The ban has been lifted in a few states and the gooseberry is starting to gain some popularity among Americans.

Gooseberries belong to the gooseberry family (*Grossulariaceae*). They are true berries, each about the size of a hazelnut and yellowish-green to purple in colour. They are easy to grow, but prefer relatively cool climates and moist, well-drained soils to produce berries that are sweet and deliciously juicy when left on the bush to ripen fully. Small, bell-shaped flowers appear on the prickly bushes in late spring, and the gooseberries are ready for picking in the middle of summer. It is a good idea to thin the berries at the beginning of summer before they ripen: under-ripe berries can be used to make jams, tarts and sauces, leaving the rest to grow bigger and sweeter.

With their high vitamin C content and plenty of phenolic acids and anthocyanins, gooseberries are powerful antioxidants that support the immune defence system against infectious disease and have anti-inflammatory properties. They are good for the heart, circulation and nervous system, and may also help the immune system deal with mutant and cancerous cell development. Gooseberries are low in calories, high in fibre and very high in vitamin C. They also contain vitamin A and B-complex vitamins, and a number of minerals important for health, especially potassium, copper and manganese.

(RED) GRAPE *Vitis vinifera*

Botanically, grapes are true berries. They originate from the southern shores of the Caspian Sea but are now grown throughout the temperate and semi-tropical regions of the world. Grapes grow in large clusters from vigorous climbing vines and different varieties produce grapes that range from black through red, pink, yellow to green and almost white. The original grape berries were much smaller than the varieties we eat today and had bigger seeds and tougher skins. All grapes are healthy to eat but only red grapes contain the most powerful antioxidants.

The ancient Essenes cultivated grapes extensively around the Dead Sea, and knowledge of their qualities soon spread along the North African coast and around the Mediterranean countries. Natural yeast causing fermentation of overripe grapes led to the first production of wine, and the ancient Egyptians, Greeks, Phoenicians and Romans also grew grapes for food, wine and medicine.

HABITAT

Wild grapes now grow in many diverse places such as deserts, tropical regions, on the edges of temperate forests, pine woods and dry coastal areas. They are a favourite food for many wild birds and animals.

Vitis vinifera is the grape we know from gardens and greenhouses. It is a deciduous, fast-growing climber, preferring a sheltered, southwest-facing site, perhaps against a wall. The deep purple grapes ripen and are ready to eat from late summer into the autumn. They love heat and sun, and so are easiest to grow sheltered under glass in a temperate climate.

Grapes can survive some frost and grow as far north as Canada, Scandinavia and Russia, and as far south as Chile, South Africa and New Zealand. The top 10 commercial producers of grapes today are Italy, China, the United States, France, Spain, Turkey, Iran, Argentina, Chile and India.

PHYTONUTRIENTS
Analysis reveals that 100g/3½oz of red grapes provide 66 calories, and contain 2% protein, 1% fat, 94% carbohydrate and 3% fibre, vitamins C, K, B1, B2 and B6, iron, manganese and potassium. They are rich in antioxidants, notably resveratrol, anthocyanins, phenols, tannins, quercetin and flavonols.

QUALITIES
Records of grape cures go back 8,000 years. They were first mentioned in the Essene records, but are also referred to in Greek and Roman history, and during the Middle Ages grape cures were used in southern France, northern Italy, the south of Spain and some parts of North Africa. The famous medieval medical school of Salerno, Italy, described hundreds of cases cured by the consumption of grapes.

Today, the grape cure is practised by naturopaths as an effective detox, best undertaken in the early autumn when the grapes are abundant and before the weather gets too cold. It is very cleansing, helps to restore and rebuild body cells and stores up vitality for the winter months.

THE NINE-DAY GRAPE CURE
Use organic, seedless grapes and organic grape juice.
- For three days, eat only grapes – as many as you like – and drink only water.
- For the next three days, drink only water and diluted grape juice. Drink at least 2l/70fl oz/8½ cups of fluid per day.
- For the remaining three days, eat only grapes again, as many as you like, and drink only water. Ensure you get plenty of rest, fresh air and sunshine during the cure.
- To keep your gums in good condition, exercise them by chewing sunflower seeds every day.

After the cure, you should feel wonderfully refreshed and, most likely, will have lost some weight. This is the time to adopt a healthier lifestyle, with time and space for rest and play, fresh air and exercise. You must make sure that you eat plenty of fresh fruit and vegetables, and only small amounts of meat, dairy and sugar.

Resveratrol, a polyphenol that is found mainly in red grape skin and seeds, has been shown to aid fat metabolism and to inhibit the oxidation of low-density lipoproteins into the more health-challenging high-density form, thus lowering blood cholesterol levels. This process also helps prevent the aggregation of platelets and the formation of blood clots, which may explain the so-called 'French Paradox' that has puzzled nutritionists for a number of years. Researchers noted that as a nation, the French tend to eat a rich diet, often smoke cigarettes and regularly drink wine and liqueurs, yet they have a lower incidence of heart disease than the rest of Europe. This is thought to be because they drink red wine containing polyphenols, which protect blood vessels from damage and prevent blood vessel constriction. The alcohol content of the wine also helps to reduce blood clot formation and increases vasodilation.

Grapeseed oil is extracted from the crushed seeds and has a clean, light flavour, making it good for use in salad dressings and in baking, cosmetics and therapeutics. It is polyunsaturated, containing plenty of omega oils, and has a high content of vitamin E and phytosterols.

Grapes and grape juice can be beneficial in preventing and treating cancer, blood clots, high blood pressure, degenerative nerve disorders and Alzheimer's disease.

AVAILABILITY AND STORAGE
If you have the right garden conditions, try growing your own grapes. Otherwise, they are easy to buy fresh, or dried as raisins, as well as in food products and drinks. Rinse whole bunches and store in a bowl at room temperature to bring out the flavour. Refrigerate or freeze rinsed, dry grapes in resealable bags (see page 15).

CULINARY USES
Grapes are added to a wide range of dishes and salads to give flavour, fragrance and colour. They are good as a snack as well as in juices, jellies, jams, vinegars, wine, and in grapeseed extract and oil.

VARIETIES
There are hundreds of varieties of red grapes, which are divided into 'table' and 'wine' types, with or without seeds. Famous table varieties include 'Black Rose',

'Valencia', 'Black Corinth' (producing small grapes that are dried as currants), 'Black Monukka' (dried to make sweet raisins), 'Cardinal' (which are seedless) and 'Red Globe'. Famous wine-making varieties include 'Comtessa', 'Pinot Noir', 'Cabernet Sauvignon', 'Merlot', 'Lambrusco' and 'Muscat'.

Honeyberry *Lonicera caerulea*

This lesser-known berry, also known as blue-berried honeysuckle or sweetberry honeysuckle, is one of the few edible species produced by the honeysuckle family. Native to Siberia, northern China and northern Japan, it is very hardy and easy to grow. A small shrub, about 1–2m/3–6ft tall, it likes rich soil and full sun, but can also withstand very cold temperatures down to −40°C (−40°F). Yellowish-white flowers appear in late winter or early spring, followed by the berries. Once ripe, honeyberries turn blue with a pale waxy coating and their pulp changes colour from green to purplish red. Honeyberries are usually ready to harvest in the early summer, often before or around the same time as strawberries, making them one of the first crops of the season. They are best planted in pairs or groups to increase pollination and fruit yield.

Honeyberries taste very similar to blueberries, but with a hint of blackcurrant in their flavour. They also have the same colour skin as blueberries, but are much more elongated in shape and noticeably larger. They have a very thin skin that almost melts in the mouth, and taste delicious fresh or frozen, and in jams, jellies, juices, smoothies, yogurt, sauces and ice creams.

Honeyberries contain high levels of anthocyanins, flavonoids, vitamin C, calcium, fibre and omega oils. In Japan, where the honeyberry is known as *haskap*, one brand of juice is marketed optimistically as a 'remedy for eternal youth and longevity'. Although this is obviously an unrealistic claim, modern research does suggest that honeyberries can offer many health benefits to those who consume them: they can help to lower blood pressure and are beneficial to the heart, circulation and digestion. They can also help to support the immune system in fighting infection and cancer, and their strong antioxidant qualities make them useful in dealing with inflammation.

(Red) Huckleberry *Vaccinium parvifolium*

The red huckleberry, which is also sometimes known as red bilberry and red whortleberry, is native to western North America and British Columbia. It is found in cool, shady areas, often growing on old decaying wood stumps and logs in moist pine forests and wetlands from sea level up to 1,500m/4,920ft.

The red huckleberry is a deciduous shrub belonging to the heather family (*Ericaceae*). It grows up to 4m/13ft high with small, bright-green leaves alternating on thin, crooked branches. In the spring, bell-shaped, pink flowers hang from the boughs and are gradually replaced by small, bright red berries that ripen in the summer and stay on the branches into the winter. Red huckleberries are easily harvested by simply brushing them into a basket (instead of picking them off the twigs individually).

For generations, red huckleberry was an important year-round source of food for many Native Americans who would eat them fresh, or pressed into cakes and dried for the winter. They were also (and are still) an important food source for birds and other wildlife. Nowadays, red huckleberries are available fresh, frozen or tinned, and can be dried, mashed or pressed for juice. Though quite tart, they are excellent in smoothies, jams, pies and desserts, as a relish or made into wine.

Rich in vitamin C, sugars, fibre and minerals, as well as flavonoids and tannins, red huckleberries have a strong antioxidant effect and are also mildly astringent and diuretic. The juice of the berries can be used as a gargle for sore throats, as a mouthwash and also as an appetite stimulant that helps keep blood sugar stable.

Indian Gooseberry/Amla
Emblica officinalis (syn. *Phyllanthus emblica*)

The Indian gooseberry is also known as amla, from the Sanskrit word *amalika*, meaning 'sour juice of the fruit', an apt description of the berry's taste, which is sour, bitter and astringent. However, this berry is highly valued by nutritionists and practitioners of Ayurvedic medicine, and is commonly eaten as a pickle in India, where it is a very important source of vitamin C. It is also the main ingredient in a 5,000-year-old rejuvenating herbal tonic known as *chayavan prash*, recorded in early Ayurvedic medical texts and still used today.

Indian gooseberries belong to the leaf flower family (*Phyllanthaceae*) and grow on a deciduous tree that has a crooked trunk and feathery, light green leaves closely set along its spreading branches. It grows wild in the forests and coastal regions of India and Kashmir. The flowers that precede the berries are lime green to pale yellow in colour and, when ripe in the autumn, the juicy berries are also light green, round, smooth and hard with six vertical furrows or stripes, resembling round gooseberries.

Raw amla is extremely rich in easily absorbable vitamin C, and medical studies suggest that amla has antiviral, as well as antibacterial and antifungal properties. In Ayurvedic medicine, it is thought of as a good liver stimulant with cooling, gently laxative properties. Research from Japan suggests that amla is a potent scavenger of free radicals, thus enhancing cellular regeneration during cancer treatment. It also acts as an immune booster against colds, influenza and chronic lung disease such as tuberculosis. Some recent studies have shown that it may have potential for lowering blood cholesterol and helping to balance blood sugar levels in diabetes.

Indian gooseberries can be eaten raw, cooked, pickled with salt, oil and spices, or soaked in syrup.

Jujube/Chinese Date *Ziziphus jujuba*

A shrub of the buckthorn family (*Rhamnaceae*), the jujube originated in China, where it has been cultivated for over 4,000 years. It is now grown throughout southern Asia, India, the Korean peninsula and southeastern Europe.

The deciduous tree can grow 5–10m/16–33ft high, and has thorny branches and shiny green leaves. The flowers are small with five tiny, lime-green petals. The jujube berry is oval and 2–3cm/¾–1¼in across and changes from green to orange to red while maturing. Before fully ripe it has a consistency and flavour similar to that of an apple. The fully ripe berry turns dark red to almost black, and becomes soft and wrinkled, until it resembles a small date (hence it is also known by the names red date and Chinese date). There is a single, small, hard stone inside, so in botanical terms the jujube berry is a drupe.

Fresh and candied berries are popular as snack foods, and dried jujubes are good in desserts and drinks. For cooking in recipes, look for pitted, dried jujubes and rinse or soak before use. Tea bags and juices are available in health food stores and Chinese food stores.

A jujube decoction (made by simmering the berries in water for 5–10 minutes) can be used to treat sore throats and colds, and the pulp of the fruit can be applied to cuts and wounds and used as a skin cleanser, to improve skin colour and tone. In Arabian traditional medicine, the jujube was said to cure coughs, resolve lung complaints, soothe internal organs and reduce water retention. Dried ripe jujube berries also work as a mild laxative. In India and Pakistan, they are used as a blood cleanser, a tonic and a general preventer of disease.

In Chinese medicine, the jujube is prescribed to relieve stress and increase stamina. It is thought of as a *qi* tonic and is said to aid liver function and help recovery from hepatitis and other liver diseases. It is also used to relieve the emotional upset and debility caused by psychological illness, and its mild sedative action makes it useful for treating nervousness, restlessness and irritability. The jujube berry is rich in vitamins A, C and B2, and in the minerals calcium, phosphorus and iron. It also contains saponins, flavonoids and mucilage.

Juniper *Juniperus communis*

The juniper bush is the world's most widely distributed member of the cypress family (*Cupressaceae*). It can be found from the Arctic, through the cooler regions of Scandinavia, Europe and America to the mountains of Central America, Africa and Asia to Korea and Japan. Its distribution is closely related to the routes followed by migratory birds and to the pattern of ice distribution in the last Ice Age.

The common juniper comes in many shapes and sizes – dense shrubs, creeping evergreens, even small trees – but always sports the same sharp, blue-green needles. Juniper berries are actually small fleshy cones that can take over two years to ripen from green to dark purple. They are well known for adding spice and flavour to foods and drinks, notably gin, which started life as a tincture made by a Dutch herbalist, possibly following an old monastic recipe for a remedy to stimulate appetite. As with several other herbal tinctures (including vermouth), people soon forgot why they were drinking the gin! Juniper is also used as a flavouring in many beverages, bakery products, sweets, desserts and savoury dishes.

To the old-time herbalist, juniper was an important remedy for colds, fevers, coughs, indigestion, wind, rheumatic conditions and urinary tract complaints. It was also considered an effective disinfectant and treatment for bad breath. Modern medicinal uses for juniper are primarily as a diuretic and urinary antiseptic in urinary tract complaints, and as a soothing remedy for digestive problems caused by poor secretion of gastric juices. It can also be used to ease muscle pains and sore joints.

Ripe juniper berries are high in volatile oils (16%), resin, tannins and vitamin C. They should not be eaten daily, nor used as medicine for more than two weeks at a time, and should not be taken at all by pregnant or breast-feeding women, or by people suffering from chronic kidney problems (such as Bright's disease).

KIWI FRUIT / CHINESE GOOSEBERRY *Actinidia deliciosa*

The kiwi fruit, or Chinese gooseberry, is a true berry with rough brownish skin, juicy bright green or golden flesh and black edible seeds. Roughly the size of a hen's egg, it is unrelated botanically to the gooseberry family, although it does come originally from China, where it is the national fruit. Seeds were taken to New Zealand in 1904 and bore their first fruits there in 1910. With its refreshing, gooseberry-like taste, the berry became increasingly popular, and New Zealand began exporting to the United States in the 1950s. With the Cold War in full swing, however, anything Chinese was regarded with suspicion, so New Zealand growers had the idea of renaming it 'kiwi fruit' after the round, furry, brown flightless bird that is their national symbol (and could be said to resemble a Chinese gooseberry). 'Kiwi' is also a colloquial name for New Zealanders.

HABITAT
The kiwi fruit belongs to the Chinese goosberry family (*Actinidiaceae*) and are native to southern China. Grown in mainly mountainous areas, they thrive in strong sunshine yet can withstand frost at −30°C (−22°F). The plants are dioecious, meaning individual plants are male or female, though only the female plants bear fruit. Italy is now the world leader of commercial kiwi fruit production, followed by China, New Zealand,

Australia, Chile, Greece, Japan and the United States. New Zealand has introduced the brand name 'Zespri' as a way to distinguish the real 'Kiwi' kiwi fruit from the rest.

PHYTONUTRIENTS
Analysis reveals that 100g/3½oz of kiwi fruit provide 58 calories, and contain 8% protein, 8% fat, 72% carbohydrate and 12% fibre. They are very high in vitamin C (74% RDA) and rich in vitamins B6, E and K, potassium and magnesium. They also contain chlorophyll, flavonoids, actinidin, calcium oxalate and carotenoids beta-carotene, lutein and zeaxanthin (especially in the gold kiwi fruit). The abundant edible seeds have a high omega-3 fatty acid content.

NOTE
- Some people are allergic to the actinidin and calcium oxalate in kiwi fruit and may suffer from an itchy, sore mouth and wheezing if they eat it. People who are allergic to latex, avocado, banana, papaya and pineapple are more likely to be allergic to kiwi fruit.

QUALITIES
Kiwi fruit stimulate the immune system and are good for the skin and mucous membranes, and because of their high fibre content, they can be effective against constipation. A kiwi a day can help prevent or relieve high blood pressure and other cardiovascular problems, and can also help to improve sleep and relaxation.

The actinidin in kiwi fruit is a protein-dissolving enzyme that can aid digestion in the same way as papaya and pineapple. It also acts as a blood thinner, reducing platelet aggregation, blood fat levels and the risk of blood clots. Actinidin is also used to tenderize meat before cooking. The downside to actinidin is that it dissolves protein in dairy and gelatin, making kiwi fruit hard to use in many desserts, although the popular New Zealand version of pavlova consists of meringue and whipped cream topped with fresh kiwi slices.

AVAILABILITY AND STORAGE
Kiwi fruit are readily available in supermarkets and stores, but you can also try and grow your own. Take some seeds from a ripe kiwi fruit and dry them on kitchen paper. Plant the seeds in a little compost and grow in containers in a greenhouse or conservatory or, if the climate is warm and sunny enough, on a terrace.

If kept cool, unripe kiwi fruit can be stored for up to six months. At room temperature, out of direct sunlight, they will normally keep for one or two weeks. They ripen faster in a paper bag with an apple, pear or banana that emits ethylene gas.

CULINARY USES

Kiwi fruit are delicious eaten just as they are or sliced into salads, on breakfast cereals, cakes and desserts, or blended into juices and smoothies. A fun way to eat a kiwi is to halve it and serve in an egg cup so the flesh can be scooped out with a teaspoon.

VARIETIES

The Golden Kiwi/Zespri Gold has smooth, edible skin, golden-yellow flesh and a more tropical flavour than the green kiwi fruit. There is also a red variety available now in which the fruit reveals a striking red central star on a golden background.

Lingonberry *Vaccinium vitis-idaea*

Lingonberries, also known as cowberries, foxberries, partridgeberries, redberries and at least 20 other common names, are native to the Arctic tundra. The low, evergreen, bushy plants, belonging to the heather family (*Ericaceae*), have light brown stems and small, oval leaves. They flower in early summer, producing tiny bell-shaped, white or pale pink flowers that turn into small, round, bright red berries that become ripe and ready for picking from late summer into the autumn.

The bushes keep their leaves all through winter and are extremely hardy, tolerating very low temperatures down to −40°C (−40°F). They prefer cool summers too, with plenty of shade and a moist and acidic, nutrient-poor soil. The name 'lingonberry' comes from the Swedish name, *lingon*, and they are commonly found in the Scandinavian mountains and forests, the Arctic tundra and the northern wildernesses of Russia, Canada and the United States.

The berries have a sharp, acidic taste and are often mistaken for cranberries, although cranberries are duller in colour, have a much sharper flavour and are more sensitive to nutrient-rich soils. In fact, lingonberries are taking over from cranberries in the wilds of Scandinavia, pushing cranberries to a shrinking habitat in the higher-lying bogs that are not reached by nutrient-rich agricultural run-off.

Traditionally, lingonberries are harvested in the wild, a favourite summer pastime in Sweden. In recent years, the bushes have become increasingly popular ornamental garden plants, admired for their strikingly bright, glossy berries and neat evergreen leaves. In the wild, lingonberries provide an important source of food for wildlife, especially birds, bears and foxes. Historically, they were also significant for indigenous people living in the remote northern wastelands who found that eating lingonberries gave protection against scurvy and could ease diarrhoea and other complaints.

Lingonberries are a good source of fibre, sugars, vitamins A, B-complex and C, and magnesium, calcium, potassium and phosphorus. They also offer many phytonutrients such as antioxidants, beta-carotene, tannins, anthocyanins, proanthocyanidin, arbutin, lignans, flavonoids, resveratrol, benzoic acid and quercetin. They may be able to mop up free radicals and prevent cells from turning cancerous while also helping the immune system deal with those that have mutated. They have also been shown to be beneficial in treating some infections, particularly of the urinary tract, and those caused by *E. coli*.

Traditionally, lingonberries were stored in water-filled jars throughout winter. These days it is probably easier to pop them in the freezer. Eat them raw, rinsed and with a little sugar, or in jams, compotes, juices or syrups, or as a main-dish accompaniment.

Loganberry *Rubus* x *loganobaccus*

A hybrid between the American blackberry and the European raspberry, the loganberry belongs to the rose family (*Rosaceae*). It is large and long, becoming a bright, deep purple when ripe. The juicy berries are ready to pick at different times from early in the season and have a sharp yet refreshing acidic flavour.

The story goes that loganberries were accidently created by a Californian horticulturist named James Harvey Logan, who wanted to improve on the existing varieties of blackberries and create a cultivar that would produce larger and juicier fruit. Logan planted two varieties of blackberry next to an old variety of raspberry. When the plants cross-pollinated, a hybrid was born. Mr Logan gathered the berries (or rather, the composite fruits) containing the seeds and planted them. The result was plants that grew vigorously and bore fruits that look like large, firm, dark reddish-purple blackberries with a fine flavour.

Since this time, many growers have made new crosses between raspberries and blackberries, but the name given to the first hybrid, created in the 1880s, remains the same. In the 1930s, a non-prickly variety was developed and loganberries have proved to be productive and easy to grow. The plants are sturdy and more frost resistant than other berries. The vines trail on the ground like dewberry vines and can grow up to 3m/10ft in one season. Old canes die after the second season, and should be cut away. Plants can self-propagate and continue to bear fruit for up to 15 years.

Loganberries can be eaten raw, juiced or cooked, and are particularly good in salads, snacks, jellies, jams, wines, syrups, pies, trifles and crumbles. They have a high vitamin C content and, since they also keep well, they were used by the British navy in the early part of the 20th century to help prevent scurvy. They are also rich in anthocyanins, ellagic acid, rutin, fibre, vitamin K, folate and manganese. As they have strong antioxidants with antiviral and antibacterial properties, loganberries may be of help in reducing the risk of cancer and in strengthening the body's immune defences.

Mulberry *Morus* spp

There are several different species of mulberry tree, belonging to the mulberry or fig family (*Moraceae*) that can be divided into three main types: the white, native to China; the black, native to the Middle Eastern lands of ancient Mesopotamia and Persia (present-day Iraq and Iran); and the red, native to North America.

Mulberries have been eaten and used as medicine since ancient times, and are mentioned in the Bible and in early Roman texts. Ovid, the Roman poet, tells the sad tale of two lovers who committed suicide under a mulberry tree, their blood turning its white berries black. The mulberry was probably introduced to northern Europe by the Roman armies, who brought the berries in their food supplies. The oldest living mulberry tree in England is thought to come from Persia and dates back to the 16th century. Native Americans have also used the mulberry tree and its red berries for food and medicine for generations.

Mulberry trees are easy to grow and can reach 10–15m/33–50ft high, depending on the species. They are self-fertilizing, and the berries are 2–3cm/ ¾–1¼in long and look like large blackberries or raspberries, which, like the mulberry, are classified botanically as composite fruits. Mulberries do not all ripen at the same time, even on the same tree, and can continue to mature over quite a long period during early autumn. They are very sweet and juicy, especially the black ones, and can be used raw, dried or frozen in juices, jams, jellies, pies, pancakes, muesli, bakes, snacks, sauces and, of course, for mulberry wine. They will only keep for a few days after picking, however, so need to be frozen or dried immediately after harvesting. The leaves of the mulberry tree are the only natural food source for silkworms.

Mulberries have a high vitamin C and iron content, and are rich in fibre, vitamins K and B2, calcium, magnesium and potassium. They also contain anthocyanins, including a dark-coloured natural dye that turns fingers orange, red, purple, blue or even black when picking the fruits. Studies have shown that eating mulberries can help to lower cholesterol and reduce high blood pressure, and they may also have a role in the management of infection, diabetes, cancer and degenerative neurological diseases.

Much of the current medical interest in mulberries relates to the fact that they are known to contain resveratrol and phyto-oestrogens. Foods containing these two components have been shown to have the potential to prevent hormone-related cancers, including some types of breast cancer, and to inhibit the growth of cancer cells. Resveratrol has also been shown to reduce oxidative stress and so may have an impact on the rate of neuronal loss in senile neurodegenerative disorders, such as Alzheimer's disease. Studies have shown that including foods high in resveratrol in the diet can protect neurons from oxidative damage and help slow cognitive decline.

Oregon grape *Mahonia aquifolium*

The Oregon grape is a popular, low-maintenance plant belonging to the barberry family (*Berberidaceae*) and is often seen in suburban hedges and gardens. There are more than 100 species and, as its common name suggests, this plant is native to the west coast of North America and is the official state flower of Oregon. It was given its name by the early pioneers who harvested the berries along the Oregon trail, but these days the plant is available from nurseries all over the world. It is drought resistant and frugal, being able to thrive in very poor soils. It is also good for wildlife: hummingbirds and bees take nectar from the flowers, and the berries are a good winter food source for birds and other wildlife. The leaves are holly-like, prickly and leathery, and the plant flowers in late spring with characteristic clusters of small yellow flowers. The berries grow in bunches and have a slightly dusty appearance, resembling dark blue grapes. They ripen in late summer, remaining on the bush in winter, and they have long featured in the lives of the Native Americans of the Pacific Northwest. Traditionally, the root has been used medicinally as an anti-inflammatory and a natural antibiotic, and as the whole plant was believed to provide protection and positive energy, it was often used in protective talismans. Adding a sprig of Oregon grape to a bunch of flowers is still thought by many to help create a positive atmosphere in gatherings and meetings, and Oregon grape wood is popular for making crucifixes.

Oregon grape berries can be quite tart and bitter, depending on how much water they contain, but like many other tart berries they become sweeter after a frost. They can be used fresh, dried or frozen, but are nicer to eat with the large seeds removed as these can be chewy. Strained through a sieve/fine-mesh strainer or a thin muslin cloth/cheesecloth, Oregon grapes make a beautiful jelly, and are also used to make wine. They can also add interest and taste to pies and stews, and may be used in recipes as a substitute for blackberries.

The main medicinal value of the Oregon grape plant is in the root, but the berries also have gentle medicinal qualities. They are useful immune boosters and are beneficial in the prevention and treatment of 'lifestyle diseases' such as heart disease and diabetes. They have a cooling effect, and can be used to ease gastritis and other digestive problems. Like many berries with beneficial effects on health, Oregon grapes are rich in vitamin C and pectin, and contain antioxidant anthocyanins. They also contain small amounts of berberine, which stimulates liver function and so can help purify the blood.

Persimmon *Diospyros* spp

Also known as Sharon fruit, date plums and kaki, persimmons are the edible fruits (berries, in botanical terms) of a number of species belonging to the ebony family (*Ebenaceae*). The Greek name *diospyros* means 'fruit of the gods', and they really do have a delicately divine taste that justifies their nickname 'nature's candy'.

The persimmon tree is quick-growing, deciduous and attractive. It can reach up to 8m/26ft in height and prefers mild climates with moderate winters and mild summers. It is one of the last trees to bloom in spring, with flowers that appear after the leaves, and fruits that ripen in the autumn, hanging off the branches long into winter, after the leaves have fallen. The most commonly produced persimmons, from *Diospyros virginiana*, are light to dark orange in colour, and vary in size. There are many other varieties native to different parts of the world, from the Americas to Asia, North Africa and Europe. The leading producers of persimmons are China, Japan, Korea, Brazil, Italy, New Zealand, Iran, Australia and Mexico, and commercial growers concentrate on just two varieties: the astringent and the non-astringent. The astringent variety is high in tannins and commonly grown in Japan. It needs to ripen fully and become jelly-soft before it is ready to eat. The non-astringent variety contains less tannin and has a crisp consistency, similar to pears and apples.

High in sugar and fibre, rich in vitamins A and C, and with a good content of vitamins E and B6, potassium, copper and manganese, persimmons contain important antioxidant flavonoids such as catechins, betulinic acid, beta-carotene, lycopene, lutein and xanthins. Catechins are known to have antibacterial and anti-inflammatory properties, and can improve capillary wall integrity, thus preventing bleeding from small blood vessels. Vitamin C helps the body resist infectious diseases and, together with the other antioxidants, helps protect body cells against deterioration and ageing.

Raspberry *Rubus idaeus* and *Rubus strigosus*

Wild raspberries are native to the forests of North America, Europe and Asia. The European and the American varieties are closely related, and most modern cultivars are hybrids of the two. The Roman armies are thought to be responsible for the spread of raspberries throughout Europe, but raspberry plant remains dating back as far as 4000 BC have been found in Switzerland.

The raspberry is really an aggregate fruit, consisting of numerous drupelets arranged around a central core. Depending on the variety, the berries ripen from early summer into the autumn. The plant belongs to the rose family (*Rosaceae*) and grows best in cooler climates as they can suffer root rot if the soil is too warm or wet. Once raspberries are established in a habitat, they can be extremely vigorous – and invasive.

The berries and leaves of the raspberry cane have long been used as food and medicine, and raspberry growing is now an international business with the top 10 commercial producers being Russia, Serbia, the USA, Poland, Germany, Ukraine, Canada, Hungary, the United Kingdom and France. The berries are fragile and keep for only a few days in the refrigerator after picking, so it is best not to rinse them until just before use. They can be enjoyed fresh, frozen or dried.

Some old pharmacopoeias refer to the ability of raspberries to strengthen the heart, and highlight their use in relieving coughs, colds and influenza. Raspberry vinegar is a tried and tested remedy against fevers, sore throats and chest complaints, and today we know that raspberries contain important polyphenols, anthocyanins and ellagic acid that have significant anti-inflammatory, antibacterial and antioxidant effects. They can also help to decrease the rate of cancer cell proliferation and may play a role in slowing the processes of age-related disease. Oil extracts from raspberry seeds can be used for skin healing and as moisturizers because of their vitamin E and omega fatty acid content.

Raspberries are high in protein, sugars and fibre, and are also rich in vitamins A, C, B1, B2, B3 and K, and minerals iron, calcium, potassium, manganese and copper. They are also rich in citric acid, malic acid, pectin, ellagic tannins, catechins, kaempferol and salicylic acid. This combination of phytochemicals, vitamins and minerals helps the body to counter inflammation, develop resistance against infection, metabolize carbohydrates, protein and fats, control heart rate and blood pressure, and keep on producing healthy red blood cells. Like most other berries, raspberries have a low glycaemic index due to their xylitol content. Xylitol is a low-calorie sugar that is absorbed slowly and so may be helpful in the management of diabetes.

Redcurrant *Ribes rubrum*

Wild redcurrants are native to Europe, Asia and North America and classed as members of the gooseberry family (*Grossulariaceae*). The first large-berried varieties were cultivated in the 17th century by French and Belgian growers and were taken to America by European settlers.

Easy to grow and very low maintenance, the redcurrant bush is just over 1m/3ft tall and prefers well-drained but moist, non-acidic soil and full sunlight or light shade.

Redcurrants thrive in woodland, hedges and domestic gardens, but shouldn't be planted near pine trees as they can harbour the fungal disease white pine blister rust. This susceptibility led to them and other *Ribes* species being banned from the US in the 1920s until recently (although they were themselves victims as much as hosts of the disease).

Redcurrants are self-fertilizing and the bushes start bearing fruit when they are three to four years old. The flowers are small and yellow-green, appearing in small hanging clusters in the spring, and maturing during the summer into small bunches of bright red, translucent berries with up to 10 in each bunch. The berries are very popular with birds so if you want to keep the crop for yourself, they should be protected with netting. Alternatively, use them as a bribe to deter birds from eating other fruits and berries in the garden.

Redcurrants contain four times as much vitamin C as oranges, which explains their tart taste. They are refreshing to eat raw, rinsed and with a little sugar. They are also excellent in jams, jellies, condiments, preserves, pies, juices, syrups and wine.

Redcurrants are fat-free, low-calorie, high-fibre berries that are rich in vitamins C and K, and contain good amounts of iron, potassium, copper and manganese, and antioxidant anthocyanins. The vitamin C facilitates iron absorption and is a vital antioxidant that can help the immune system to fight disease and heal damaged tissues.

Rose hip *Rosa canina, Rosa rugosa* and spp

The wild rose species, belonging to the rose family (*Rosaceae*), include the dog rose and the beach rose, and are commonly found growing alongside streams and in hedgerows and woods throughout Europe, America, North Africa and southwest Asia. There are over 100 different species, varying from low bushes to large shrubs, but all have one thing in common: small, sharp thorns, which enable the wild rose to climb up through hedges, walls and trees. The wild rose's leaves consist of five or seven leaflets and its delicate flowers vary from almost white to pale pink to deep red or purple. The flowers mature into oval, orange or red hips from late summer into the autumn. Rose hips are full of seeds and, although we think of them as berries, they are more properly defined as fleshy pseudofruits.

Valued as a source of nutrition and medicine for centuries, wild rose hips are easy to find. Rose hips can be cooked to make delicious syrups, jellies and jams, or infused as a refreshing tisane, but always filter to eliminate any seed hairs. Rose hip juice is claimed to have 20 times more vitamin C than orange juice and is highly regarded as a tonic. Eaten raw, they have an intense apple-like flavour, and are excellent served as a snack or in salads, or can be baked in breads.

The name 'dog rose' is thought to refer to the plant's use in past centuries to treat bites from rabid dogs. Rose hips also have a long tradition of being taken to relieve respiratory and digestive conditions. As one of today's natural remedies, rose hips are thought to help improve immunity to infections, boost energy levels, maintain the health of mucous membranes, enhance wound healing and help prevent cardiovascular disease and the development of cancer cells. Recent studies show that rose hips may also be useful in the treatment of osteoarthritis, helping to relieve pain from sore and inflamed joints.

Taking rose hips regularly has been shown to lower systolic blood pressure and regulate blood sugar and cholesterol levels, which could significantly reduce cardiovascular risk in obese people and those suffering from diabetes. As well as vitamin C, rose hips contain carotenoids, tannins, pectins and vitamins A, B1 and B2.

WARNING

- The hairs around the seeds can cause irritation and should not be eaten. Remove the seeds and rinse the hips well before eating raw. Use whole hips in tisanes.

Rowan *Sorbus* spp

The rowan tree belongs to the rose family (*Rosaceae*) and is native to cool regions of the Northern Hemisphere and also known as mountain ash. It is one of the hardiest European trees, and can grow in very poor soil as long as it is well drained. Found in woods, borders and on rocky hillsides, in sun or partial shade, this elegant tree turns bright red in the autumn, and the name 'rowan' is thought to derive from this fact. Once considered a magical tree, the rowan also has a long list of other names throughout the world, many of which can be linked to the mythology and folklore surrounding it.

The tree is deciduous and its leaves consist of between 10 and 35 small leaflets. The flowers are creamy white and arranged in dense clusters that appear in the spring and go on to develop into small pomes (the botanical term for rowan berries) over the summer into autumn. These are mostly bright orange or red, but can be pink, yellow or white in some species. Birds love to eat the soft, juicy and waxy berries that stay on the tree throughout the winter, but to the human palate they taste tart, bitter and mealy (although the taste becomes gentler after they have had frost).

Rowan berries can be eaten raw or cooked and make excellent, slightly bitter jellies, jams and preserves. They taste especially good when combined with apples or pears, and can also be used to make or flavour liqueurs, wines and cordials.

In traditional medicine, rowan berries have been used to treat constipation, gout, kidney disease, arthritis and diabetes. As the berries are astringent and antibiotic, small amounts of rowan juice can be beneficial as a gargle to treat sore throats, hoarseness and tonsillitis. They are rich in fibre, iron and vitamin C, and contain good amounts of fructose, vitamins A, K and B3, folate, potassium, calcium, magnesium, carotenoids, tannins and parasorbic acid. Parasorbic acid is strongest in the fresh berries and can cause local irritation and diarrhoea, but it becomes less powerful during drying and is fully destroyed by cooking, which turns it into the more benign sorbic acid.

Salmonberry *Rubus spectabilis*

A beautiful thicket-forming shrub, belonging to the rose family (*Rosaceae*) and widely grown for its pretty purple flowers, salmonberry is native to the west coast of North America, but has also become naturalized in Europe. It is found in damp forests, alongside streams and in coastal areas, thriving particularly well under red alder trees. Salmonberries are also known as Alaska berries and grow in abundance on Raspberry Island in Alaska. They were once an important source of food to Native Americans, and (as the name suggests) were eaten with salmon.

The perennial plant grows 1–4m/3–13ft tall and flowers from early spring to early summer. The berries, which look like large yellow, orange and red raspberries, ripen individually from early summer into autumn and, like raspberries, are aggregate fruits made up of drupelets that can be pulled away from a central core. Vibrant, glossy and delicate, they have a sweet, slightly sour taste, and are good eaten raw or in jams, jellies, wine and smoothies. Because of their high water content, they are not easy to dry and deteriorate rapidly after picking, so they should be used immediately or frozen.

The salmonberry is rich in glucose, fructose, fibre and vitamins A, C, E and K. Its high vitamin C content gives it antioxidant and immunostimulant properties that can protect against infections, and vitamin A promotes healthy eyesight and skin.

Sea-buckthorn *Hippophae rhamnoides*

There are six species of sea-buckthorn, belonging to the oleaster family (*Elaeagnaceae*), native to Europe and Asia. *Hippophae rhamnoides* is by far the most widespread. It thrives in sunny, dry areas and can tolerate the salty soil and air along sea coasts where there is little competition from other plants. Despite its name, sea-buckthorn can also survive at altitude – even above the tree line.

A deciduous shrub with dense, thorny branches and distinct pale, silvery-green, long, thin leaves, the sea-buckthorn exists as both male and female plants. The male produces flowers and pollen in the spring, and the female produces tight clusters of orange, pea-size, soft, juicy berries all through the autumn. These are difficult to pick without squashing because they are arranged so densely on branches covered in sharp thorns. The easiest way to harvest sea-buckthorn is to cut the whole ends off the twigs with secateurs and then freeze them. Once frozen, the berries can be shaken off as required.

Sea-buckthorns have become popular as edible garden shrubs and can be planted to create impenetrable hedges and windbreaks. The berries stay on the branches all winter, providing an important winter food source for birds and also a welcome splash of garden colour. They can be eaten raw (after freezing to reduce their bitterness) or cooked, and go especially well with carrot and beetroot/beet in juices and smoothies. They are also used commercially to make confectionery, jams, syrups, herb teas, liqueurs, supplements and herbal products.

The exceptionally high content of vital vitamins, minerals and oils in sea-buckthorn berries has generated much interest among health professionals, and the fresh-pressed juice can be used to treat colds and influenza, fevers, inflammations and general health problems related to inadequate nutrition and a poor lifestyle. Sea-buckthorn berries are undergoing research to examine if they are capable of halting or reversing the cell mutations that can lead to cancer. The berries can also be used to treat skin conditions such as radiation-induced dermatitis, wounds, burns and premature ageing.

Overall, sea-buckthorn berries can be regarded as near-perfect natural food supplements, rich in vitamins C, A, E and B-complex, and minerals potassium, iron, calcium, magnesium, phosphorus, zinc, copper, manganese and selenium. They also contain plenty of protein, fats and omega oils, flavonoids and carotene, which makes them a valuable source of nutrition for people living or travelling in remote areas.

Seagrape *Coccoloba uvifera*

Seagrape is a sprawling evergreen shrub and member of the buckwheat family (*Polygonaceae*), native to coastal regions throughout South America and the Caribbean and naturalized in Mediterranean countries. The plant prefers full sun or light shade, and is highly tolerant of salt and wind so it is often used to stabilize beach margins. As it is easy to grow, it is also cultivated as an ornamental shrub.

The leaves are very recognizable because of their prominent red veins, and the flowers are small, white and fragrant, growing in bunches in late spring to early summer. Male and female flowers grow on separate plants so in order for the 'grapes' to develop it is necessary to grow more than one plant to ensure cross-pollination by bees and other insects. Seagrape berries form large clusters and are round or pear-shaped, ranging in colour from almost white to dark purple. The flesh surrounds a single, large seed, so in botanical terms they are classified as drupes. Unlike true grapes, they don't all ripen simultaneously and usually drop from the tree when ready to eat.

Seagrapes are slightly acidic, sweet and tasty to eat raw or cooked in jams, jellies, juices, wine and vinegar. The juice can be used to treat digestive problems and to strengthen the immune system, and it is rich in anthocyanins, carotenes, vitamins A, C, K and B-complex, iron, potassium, manganese and copper.

Serviceberry *Amelanchier* spp

The serviceberry is a shrub belonging to the rose family (*Rosaceae*) and is native to the temperate regions of the Northern Hemisphere. It grows in open woods, along streams and roads, in swamps and bogs, and on rocky mountainsides. It is also popular as an ornamental shrub because of its clusters of delicate white flowers, pale grey bark and beautiful autumn colours. The flowers appear on the shrub in the middle of spring, followed in the summer by red to purple or black berries, or pomes, containing up to five very small seeds that taste of almonds. The pomes can last until the first frost, and all 25 species are edible.

Serviceberries (or Saskatoon or juneberries as they are also known) were a major food source for the native peoples of the American prairies who used to sun- or smoke-dry them for eating and for use as a food flavouring. European settlers also learnt to use them in cooking in order to prevent various malnutrition problems such as scurvy. In culinary terms, serviceberries resemble blueberries having a sweet, pleasant flavour, and can be eaten fresh as snacks, in salads, juices and smoothies, and go well with muesli and yogurt. They are easy to freeze or dry, and are also delicious cooked in pancakes, muffins and pies, and in jams and jellies.

Traditionally, serviceberry juice was used to treat stomach complaints and to make eye and ear drops. The berries are a rich source of flavonoids with high antioxidant capacities, making them potentially important in the prevention and treatment of many chronic degenerative diseases. As well as fibre and protein, serviceberries also contain significant amounts of calcium, magnesium, potassium, zinc, iron, carotene, vitamins A, C, E and B2 and folate.

Sloe *Prunus spinosa*

Sloes are the berries of the blackthorn tree, a large deciduous shrub or small tree with dark grey or black bark and dense, spiny branches. The blackthorn is easy to confuse with the cherry plum tree but is more shrub-like, with narrower leaves and very different berries: sloes are black with an extremely tart, astringent taste, while cherry plums are yellow or red with a taste and texture similar to greengages. Blackthorn likes a sunny position and can thrive in almost any soil, apart from acid peat. Traditionally, it was planted to make cattle-proof hedges, and it is still often found in hedgerows and at the edges of fields, forests, parks and common land.

Creamy-white blackthorn flowers are some of the earliest blossoms of the year and appear in spring before the leaves come out. The berries are black drupes with one large seed and a waxy, pale blue, dusty complexion. They ripen in autumn and are usually harvested after the first frost to bring out their sweetness. The berries remain on the trees long after the leaves have fallen, until the birds have eaten them all.

Resembling small damsons with their dark skin and yellow flesh, sloes are almost inedible raw unless they have been frozen. In preserves, jams, jellies or chutneys, however, they have an intense plum taste, and make an interesting addition to pies and sponge cakes. They are also used to make Sloe Gin (see page 222), liqueurs, syrups and vinegars. Sloes preserved in vinegar resemble Japanese *umeboshi*, the extremely tart and salty plum dish often eaten (in small quantities) with rice.

Sloe syrup is a traditional flu remedy, and the berries have also been used to treat diarrhoea, relieve muscle cramps, improve digestion and lessen fever. Modern research offers some support for these uses as it has shown sloe to have a significant antibacterial effect.

Sloes are high in vitamin C, and contain antioxidant anthocyanins as well as important minerals, including calcium, magnesium and potassium. They are also high in tannins. The seed contains hydrogen cyanide, the chemical responsible for the characteristic flavour of bitter almonds. In small quantities, this phytochemical stimulates respiration and digestion, and is also thought to inhibit cancer cell growth. In excess, however, it is poisonous, so avoid eating the seeds if they are too bitter.

STRAWBERRY *Fragaria x ananassa* and spp

'Doubtless God could have made a better berry, but doubtless God never did,' wrote Dr William Butler more than four centuries ago. Most people would still agree with him: strawberries are popular all over the world for their refreshing flavour and cheerful appearance.

Botanically the strawberry belongs to the rose family (*Rosaceae*) and is neither a berry nor a fruit; it is an aggregate fruit with the seeds scattered in the skin. In ancient Rome, strawberries were seen as a cure-all and were used against everything, from fevers and fainting to inflammation and diseases of the blood, spleen and liver.

Traditionally, straw was applied as a mulch around cultivated strawberry plants in order to prevent the berries from lying directly on the ground and spoiling, hence the name 'strawberry'.

HABITAT

The wild strawberry is native to most countries in the world, except Africa, Australia and New Zealand. Long admired for its sweet flavour, the tiny woodland strawberry was being cultivated in the royal gardens of France by the 14th century, and by the 15th century, strawberry cultivation was being introduced into many of the European courts and gardens. Today, strawberries are grown in all of the world's temperate zones. The top 10 producers are the United States (more than a million tonnes a year), Turkey, Spain, Egypt, South Korea, Mexico, Japan, Poland, Germany and Russia.

PHYTONUTRIENTS

Analysis reveals that 100g/3½oz of fresh strawberries provide 33 calories, and contain 10% protein, 3% fat, 73% carbohydrate and 14% fibre. They are rich in vitamin C (96% RDA), folate (10% RDA), vitamins B1, B2, B3, B5 and B6, biotin, potassium, magnesium, iron, copper, manganese and iodine. They also contain ellagic acid, flavonoids and carotenoids lutein and zeaxanthin.

QUALITIES

Over the years, much research has gone into finding out if, how and why strawberries are not just tasty but also so nutritious. Research evidence supports their ability to strengthen the body's inherent self-healing capacity, and suggests that they can lower the risk of some of the most common killers of our time, including cardiovascular disease and cancer. Their cholesterol-lowering effect has been proven beyond doubt, and research has also shown a positive effect on skin disorders, gastrointestinal problems and chronic inflammation.

The impressively high vitamin C, ellagic acid and flavonoid content of strawberries makes them powerful antioxidants and immune boosters, and they are also helpful in the prevention of cataracts. Ellagic acid has been shown to suppress the growth of cancer cells and, together with the rest of the antioxidants in strawberries, neutralizes the negative effects of free radicals. Ellagic acid and flavonoids also counteract the effect of low-density lipoproteins (LDLs) in the blood, which can cause plaque to build up in the arteries.

Eating a small portion of strawberries each day can help to reduce symptoms of auto-immune diseases, including lupus and arthritis, although some people with arthritis find strawberries hard to digest and discover that they can aggravate symptoms.

Strawberries contain chemicals that protect against exposure to the sun. A team of Italian and Spanish scientists exposed samples of human skin-cell cultures to doses of ultraviolet light equivalent to 90 minutes of midday sun. The samples that had received the strawberry extract suffered less cell damage than the control group, which had not. This is believed to be due to the anthocyanin pigments, which give strawberries and other berries their red colour. Wild strawberries ripen in early summer, thus giving natural protection when the sun is at its strongest.

As if all that was not enough, strawberries are also one of the most delicious and versatile berries in the world. Eat them raw when they are in season and frozen when not. What could be a more delicious way to ensure good health?

WARNING

- Some people are allergic to strawberries and may experience hayfever-like symptoms when eating them. The allergen is thought to be in the fruit's red pigment, so they may find that white strawberries are better tolerated.

AVAILABILITY AND STORAGE

Pick the woodland strawberry in the wild; grow your own in garden beds or in pots; or buy them fresh, frozen or dried, or in food products and drinks. Don't rinse fresh strawberries until you are ready to eat them. Keep at room temperature for a day, or in the refrigerator for a few days in a single layer in a plastic container lined with kitchen paper. Cook, dry or freeze them if you plan to keep them for longer.

CULINARY USES

Strawberries are at their best eaten fresh, whether as a snack, on breakfast cereals, in salads, desserts and cakes, or blended into smoothies. Add frozen strawberries to juices, and make them into ice creams, yogurts, jams, drinks and preserves.

VARIETIES

The woodland strawberry is the original European strawberry. The native American strawberry was later crossed with the Chilean strawberry to create the larger modern strawberry. As its scent was likened to that of a pineapple, it was given the name *Fragaria* x *ananassa* and all the modern commercial strawberries derive from this hybrid.

There are many species, hybrids and cultivars of strawberry plants available. They are divided into two groups: the 'June-bearing' type, which only bear fruit in early summer, and the 'ever-bearing', which bear fruit all through the season. 'Earliglow' is said to be the best of the former and 'Tristar' the best of the latter, but new improved varieties come on the market all the time.

Strawberry Tree *Arbutus unedo*

Native to Mediterranean countries, the elegant strawberry tree is an evergreen shrub belonging to the heather family (*Ericaceae*). It prefers a warm, mild climate, but is also native to southwest Ireland where it was first noticed growing wild in the 19th century. Unlike most of its botanical family members, the strawberry tree prefers lime-rich soils and it has been a popular garden plant for many years. Its image also forms part of the coat-of-arms of the city of Madrid.

The strawberry tree can grow up to 10m/33ft tall and has dark green, glossy, evergreen leaves. Its white, bell-shaped flowers appear in the autumn and sit together in bunches of 10 to 30. The small, red, strawberry-like berries ripen as new flowers appear, and have a rough, gritty skin and delicate flesh, which has the texture of a tropical fruit and a pleasant sweet taste. They can be eaten raw or cooked, in pies, jams, preserves and liqueurs. Strawberry tree berries have a tendency to ferment when they have fallen from the tree, which turns their sugar content into alcohol. It is said that bears can get drunk from eating them, and so can people!

Although the strawberry tree is rarely grown as a food crop, the ripe berries do contain significant nutrients and phytochemicals, including sugars, carotenoids (including lycopene), potassium and ethyl gallate, which is a natural antibiotic. They also contain polyphenol antioxidants, which are known to help reduce the risk of degenerative diseases, cancer and cardiovascular problems, and research has shown that 100g/3½oz of strawberry tree berries can contain over 40% of the recommended daily allowance (RDA) of vitamin C.

Sumac *Rhus glabra* and *Rhus coriaria*

Smooth sumac and tanner's sumac are just two of over 250 species belonging to the *Rhus* genus of the sumac family. They will grow in any well-drained soil as long as there is plenty of sun, and can be found in thickets and hedgerows, on waste ground and by streams throughout North America, Africa, and in subtropical and temperate regions all over the world. Sumac is popular in the Middle East where it is considered an essential cooking ingredient, adding a tart, acidic flavour as well as a beautiful deep red colour.

Classified as a shrub, sumac can grow up to 3m/10ft tall and produces narrow pointed leaflets arranged in spirals. In summer, tiny lime-green flowers appear in compact cones that turn into tight clusters of velvety-soft, red berries in the autumn and stay on the tree through the winter. The berries, known as sumac bobs, are in fact drupes, and both male and female plants are required to grow fruit. Sumac is pollinated by bees, and is known to attract wildlife.

Dried sumac berries can be ground to produce a tangy, deep purple spicy powder, which is an essential ingredient in the spice mixture za'atar in Middle Eastern cuisine. It is also used as a garnish to give a lemony spark to salads, hummus, rice and kebabs as a gentler, less overpowering alternative to lemon (as indeed it was in the Middle East until the Romans introduced citrus fruits). It also lends an attractive deep red colour. Whole or powdered, sumac makes an interesting addition to pesto, soups and salad dressings. In North America there is a cool, refreshing drink called 'sumac-ade' or 'Indian lemonade', which is made by soaking the berries in boiled water for 30–40 minutes, straining, adding honey to taste and serving hot or cold with a sprig of mint. (If you try this recipe, don't let the berries boil as this releases tannins that make the drink too tart and unpleasantly astringent.)

Sumac has been used as a medicine, a spice and a dye for many centuries, especially by the Native Americans and the Arabs. Modern herbalists value the berries for their astringent, antiseptic, antifungal and antibiotic qualities, and they can also be used to prevent hyperglycaemia in type 2 diabetes, and as a gentle diuretic. They are also taken sometimes as a slimming aid, and can be used to help indigestion, calm inflammation, cool fevers and dampen period pains.

Sumac has a high content of vitamins C, B6, B1 and B2, and is also rich in fibre, potassium, calcium, magnesium, phosphorus, iron, zinc and copper. It contains anthocyanins and tannins with strong antioxidant activity, and can thus be used as a good natural antioxidant food supplement.

WARNING

- Poison sumac has white or creamy yellow berries and should be avoided.

Thimbleberry *Rubus parviflorus*

Native to North America but also found in Europe, the thimbleberry grows from sea level to altitudes of up to 2,500m/82,010ft. It prefers damp soil and is often found in open woodlands and alongside roads, tracks and streams. Thimbleberry belongs to the rose family (*Rosaceae*) and are also grown for their ornamental value; they have beautifully fragrant flowers and colourful autumn leaves.

The dense shrub grows from 1 to 2.5m/3 to 8ft tall in tight groups with canes like raspberries. However, unlike raspberry canes, thimbleberries have no thorns. The leaves are maple-shaped and large white flower blossoms appear in clusters toward the end of spring, changing into bright red berries by the end of the summer. The berries separate from the core when picked, giving a hollow fruit in the shape of a flat cap or thimble. Thimbleberry bushes are very attractive to wildlife, especially bees and butterflies, and can form an effective cover for unsightly features in the garden.

Thimbleberries, again like raspberries, are aggregate fruits with numerous drupelets around a central core, but they are larger, flatter, softer and more seedy than their better-known cousins. Their softness makes them hard to transport so they are not commonly grown commercially, but freshly picked wild or home-grown thimbleberries are delicious, with a sweet, slightly tart flavour. They can be eaten raw or dried, added to breakfast cereals and yogurts, or simply eaten on their own with a little honey. Thimbleberries also make excellent jams and jellies. High in vitamins C and A, and also containing potassium, calcium, iron and various antioxidants, they are gentle healers capable of nourishing and nurturing body tissues.

TOMATO *Solanum lycopersicum*

Belonging to the nightshade family (*Solanaceae*), tomatoes originated in South America and have spread around the world to become one of the most commonly eaten foods on the planet. More than 100 million tonnes of 7,500 varieties of tomatoes are produced and consumed worldwide each year. Cultivated by the Aztecs and the Incas as early as the 5th century BC, they were brought to Europe for the first time in the 16th century, and the word 'tomato' comes from the Aztec word *tomatl*, meaning 'swelling fruit'. The original varieties were small and yellow, and known as golden apples, or *pomi d'oro* in Italian. The French were convinced of their aphrodisiac properties and called them *pommes d'amour*.

Declared a vegetable by the US Supreme Court in 1893 (although botanically they are berries), tomatoes have become the most widely grown 'vegetable' in the world: as far north as Iceland, and as far south as the Falkland Islands. Seedlings have even been grown in space!

HABITAT

Tomatoes thrive in warm and sunny climates but they can also be grown successfully under glass. They can be divided broadly into two types according to the way they grow: bush or vine. Small bush types can be grown in pots or hanging baskets, while vine varieties need support from strings or bamboo canes. Although tomatoes are mostly grown as annuals, the tomato plant is a perennial in climates where it can survive the winter.

Although tomatoes are easy to grow from seed, they require consistent watering, feeding, training and trimming, and as much sunlight as possible (at least seven hours a day). As with all other fruits and berries, their sweetness depends on their exposure to the sun: the more sun, the higher the sugar content and the sweeter their flavour.

Varieties have been developed for the commercial market that produce tomatoes that are uniform in shape, size and colour. These are often picked when unripe, as this makes them easier to transport, and then ripened artificially with ethylene to extend their shelf life. However, this practice produces tomatoes that have a much poorer flavour and texture than those that ripen naturally on the vine.

PHYTONUTRIENTS

Analysis reveals that 100g/3½oz of tomatoes provide 20 calories, and contain 14% protein, 14% fat, 61% carbohydrate and 11% fibre. About 90% of their weight is water. They also contain vitamins A (12% RDA), C (21% RDA), E (10% RDA), B6 (10% RDA), folate (11% RDA) and vitamin K, potassium, beta-carotene, lycopene, phytosterols and flavonoids.

QUALITIES

Tomatoes are thought of as a low-calorie food because of their high water content. They are rich in lycopene, a powerful antioxidant that has been shown to protect against oxidative damage in the body. They also help protect the skin from the harmful effect of UV rays, and may offer protection against cancer (especially of the prostate and the pancreas), neurodegenerative disease, cardiovascular disease, high cholesterol and the cardiovascular problems associated with diabetes. Tomatoes can also boost resistance to infectious disease, encourage wound healing and help keep skin and mucous membranes in good condition. The potassium content of tomatoes makes them useful in cases of fluid retention and high blood pressure, and their flavonoid content makes them natural anti-inflammatories.

WARNING
- The leaves and stems of the tomato plant contain small amounts of potentially toxic alkaloids. Green, unripe tomatoes contain a low level of alkaloids but are not poisonous to eat in small amounts, for example in chutney, although they may trigger migraine attacks in susceptible individuals. They may also cause adverse reactions in those with food allergies or arthritis. All green parts of the tomato plant can be toxic to dogs and cats.

AVAILABILITY AND STORAGE
Modern cultivation techniques and transportation methods allow us to eat fresh tomatoes all through the year, but for most satisfaction (and if climate permits), try growing your own in garden beds or pots. An ever-increasingly wide selection of tomatoes can be bought fresh, dried, tinned, juiced, puréed and processed in food products and drinks. For best flavour, seek out the vine-ripened varieties. Fully ripe tomatoes keep for longer if refrigerated, but taste much better if they are brought up to room temperature for a while before eating.

CULINARY USES
Tomatoes are a versatile berry that can be enjoyed raw, cooked, juiced and pickled; on pizzas and in pasta, salads, sandwiches, salsas, soups and stews; or made into preserves. Blend whole tomatoes, including the skin, before cooking in sauces.

VARIETIES
Horticultural researchers continue to introduce new cultivars to meet consumer demand for better flavour, texture and yield. There is also great interest in increasing the range of heirloom, or heritage, varieties. Tomatoes vary in size from large beefsteak types to

dainty cherry and grape varieties, and although most tomatoes grown are classic red, they can range in colour from a pale yellow-white to purple-black.

Ugniberry *Ugni molinae* (syn. *Myrtus ugni*)

Also known as Chilean guava, the ugniberry is native to the temperate rain forests of South America, and is part of the same botanical family as guava, the myrtle family (*Myrtaceae*). It is also grown in other parts of the world, including New Zealand and Australia, where it is sometimes called 'New Zealand cranberry' or 'Tazziberry'. The ugniberry was said to be one of Queen Victoria's favourite berries as well as a popular ornamental garden plant.

As long as it receives sufficient sunlight and is not exposed to frost, an established ugniberry plant can tolerate a wide range of conditions including drought, although watering is vital until the plant becomes fully established.

The fully grown, self-fertile evergreen shrub can reach up to 2m/6ft in height and has spicy, scented leaves and small, drooping white to pale pink flowers that develop and darken into red or purple berries in the autumn. The berries resemble small round rose hips and are used extensively in Chilean cooking and to make liqueurs, jams and desserts. Their flavour is delicious and aromatic, raw or cooked, and tastes like a combination of strawberry, pineapple and apple.

Traditional healers have long used ugniberries for their medicinal properties, notably against some cancers and degenerative diseases, but more research is needed to establish the mechanisms underlying their effect. Ugniberries contain vitamins C, B6 and K, as well as folate, manganese, carotenoids and flavonoids.

Whitecurrant *Ribes rubrum*

The whitecurrant is an albino variety of the redcurrant and belongs to the gooseberry family (*Grossulariaceae*) one of the most popular varieties, 'Versailles Blanche', was first developed in France in 1843. Whitecurrants prefer a sheltered habitat, and the sweetness of their flavour depends on plenty of sun exposure.

The flowers on the whitecurrant bush are pale lime green in colour and grow in clusters. They mature into long trusses of translucent, yellow to pink, round berries that ripen early and are ready to pick in the middle of summer. Whitecurrants are smaller and sweeter than redcurrants, and should be harvested during the summer when still quite firm, and either eaten the same day, or frozen for later use. They act as a magnet for birds, however, so it is best to cover them with a fine gauge net or fruit cage.

Sweeter and less acidic than redcurrants, with a unique mild flavour, whitecurrants can be used fresh, cooked or dried, and added to cakes, tarts, casseroles, salads and vinaigrettes, or used as a tasty garnish. Cooked with a little sugar, they make a flavoursome compote to serve with yogurts and ice creams. They can also be made into preserves, wines and syrups. To preserve their flavour in an unusual jelly with a bluish-pink tint, cook whitecurrants with a little water and a tart apple. Strain, then leave to cool and set.

Whitecurrants have a high vitamin C content and are a good source of vitamins B1, B2 and B6 and minerals iron, magnesium and phosphorus. They also contain bioflavonoids (primarily in the skin and the seeds) and are rich in dietary fibre.

Whortleberry *Vaccinium uliginosum*

Also known as bog blueberry, bog bilberry and northern bilberry, the whortleberry belongs to the heather family (*Ericaceae*). It is native to the temperate northern regions and mountains of Europe, Asia, Japan and America, and is even found in the Arctic. It prefers wet, acidic soil, and flourishes in light shade or full sun.

The low, deciduous shrub has small, leathery leaves and produces pale pink, bell-shaped, hermaphrodite flowers in mid-spring. The oval berries are dark blue with light, colourless flesh and juice and have a good flavour. They are juicy and sweet, just like blueberries and bilberries, and can be eaten raw, dried or cooked.

Scientific analysis has shown that the further north whortleberries are harvested, the higher their content of powerful antioxidants and other anti-inflammatory phytochemicals. In fact, the whortleberry has a higher concentration of antioxidants than blueberries and bilberries, and the free radical scavenging capacity of these antioxidants should make whortleberries an efficient booster in the natural treatment of degenerative diseases. Research indicates that the anthocyanins in whortleberries are able to cross the blood-brain barrier, increasing neurogenesis in areas of the brain responsible for short-term memory, and positively affecting learning and memory. Other studies have demonstrated that whortleberries can cause a significant reduction in blood glucose, which has, in turn, been shown to lower the risk of dementia and other neurodegenerative conditions in diabetics.

The juice of whortleberries has been shown to prevent bacteria sticking to the bladder wall, and it can therefore be useful in the management of urinary tract infections. It is also gently antiseptic and astringent with a calming effect on the digestive system and a possible mild hypnotic action.

WARNING

- Whortleberries can cause headaches if eaten in large quantities, possibly due to fungal infestation of the raw fruit.

Wineberry *Rubus phoenicolasius*

Also known as Japanese wineberry and wine raspberry, the wineberry belongs to the rose family (*Rosaceae*) and is a species of raspberry native to northern China, Japan and Korea. It is a vigorous, invasive shrub, but it was originally introduced to Europe and America as a decorative ornamental plant. It has since become naturalized and can be found in dense thickets along the borders of fields and roads, in clearings and on waste ground in many different countries.

A perennial plant that can grow up to 3m/10ft high, it produces biennial canes with fine, hair-like, red thorns. The large leaves consist of three to five leaflets and are white underneath. The red or pink flowers appear in late spring, maturing into orange or red berries in summer and early autumn. Not true berries, but aggregate fruits consisting of numerous drupelets, wineberries are surrounded by a protective calyx with glandular hairs that give off a sticky fluid, which protects the ripening berries.

Ripe wineberries are sweet, tart and juicy, tasting like a mixture of red grapes and raspberries. They are smaller than raspberries and contain many seeds, but are still good to eat, raw or cooked. They make fine jams, jellies and wine, and are tasty additions to desserts, fruit salads, sauces and pies. They are also a good source of vitamin C, antioxidants, dietary fibre and essential minerals.

COOKING WITH BERRIES

The recipes that follow were developed to encourage people to
eat together. They are all based on fresh ingredients, with the berries
adding new colours, wonderful flavours and extra vitality to each dish.
The aim is to give you new ideas for using a variety of berries every day,
because berries offer an easy and delicious way of making your food
your medicine, and your medicine your food. All the recipes are easy
to adapt to suit different and changing dietary preferences. I myself
follow and advocate a plant-based diet, and there is a growing weight
of worldwide evidence that eating less meat is better for health, and for
the environment. If you choose to eat animal products, choose organic
as the higher up the food chain you are, the more vulnerable you become
to the effects of industrial farming practices and chemical adulteration.
I hope you will enjoy experimenting with adding berries to all sorts of
dishes and drinks. I certainly do, and I am pleased to be able to pass
what I have discovered on to you.

INTRODUCTION

My grandmother, mother and aunts were all old-school country women, each in their own way a wonderful example of robust good health based on unadulterated food and outdoor living. They taught me about growing, preserving, combining, cooking and enjoying fresh ingredients, and sparked a love of berries and wild foods that has lasted my whole life.

Later, I was privileged to be part of a mountain society where wise and frugal mountain dwellers showed me how to gather berries, fruits, mushrooms, herbs and vegetables. Their respectful attitude taught me to pay attention to where and how food is grown, and to the manner in which it is prepared, cooked and shared. In fact, the best meal I have ever enjoyed was prepared and eaten 2,000m/6,500ft up a Pyrenean mountain. It consisted mainly of freshly picked berries and mushrooms roasted over a wood fire and a drink of cool spring water.

As a result of these experiences, using food as medicine has been central to my practice as a naturopath for over 20 years, and working with patients has taught me that food, water, fresh air and exercise are powerful agents for healing and the prevention of diseases and infections. Of all the foods that enhance wellbeing, berries are perhaps the most extraordinary and versatile. They add colour, flavour and nourishment to the food we eat, and provide a foundation for long-term good health.

The recipes that follow are easy to adapt to suit different dietary preferences. I advocate a diet rich in plant foods and the use of organic produce. Here is my thinking behind choosing my key ingredients:

Meat or no meat: The weight of evidence is that reduced meat consumption is associated with better health. When you do want to eat meat, it is especially important to choose organic as the higher up the food chain you are, the more vulnerable you become to the effects of chemical adulteration of produce. Tofu, Quorn, tempeh (fermented soybeans) and seitan (fermented wheat), pulses (beans, peas and lentils), nuts and vegetables, make cheaper, and often healthier, alternatives to meat and I suggest them as alternatives to meat in many recipes.

Dairy foods: Cow's milk contains plenty of vitamins and minerals, but also contains proteins, sugars, fats and hormones that are not so easily digested by humans. In some people, cow's milk may cause digestive disorders and provoke immune reactions. Also (as all nursing mothers know), much of what is eaten by the cow passes into the milk (from stress hormones to medicines, microtoxins and nutrients), so choose organic milk and dairy products, or try non-dairy alternatives.

Plant-based dairy substitutes: Thanks to modern methods of fat emulsification, plant margarines are now free of damaging hydrogenated trans fats. Rice, soy, almond, oat, hazelnut, hemp and coconut milks are also more widely available, as are plant-based yogurts, cheeses and creams.

Eggs: I recommend free-range and organic. You can replace eggs with baking powder, vegan egg substitutes, such as No Egg, or chickpea water.

Oils: Different oils suit different purposes. Olive oil is an excellent choice for general cooking, sauces and dressings. Finer nut and seed oils are best reserved for dressings, as they do not heat well. Corn, palm and grapeseed oils are good for frying, and the properties of coconut oil make it excellent for stir-fries and, when used sparingly, for baking. Rapeseed/canola oil is also good for baking and frying.

Grains: When choosing flour, pasta and rice, whole grains are considered healthier as nothing has been removed. But children (and some people with digestive disorders) sometimes find wholemeal hard to handle. In such cases, use a mix of wholemeal and white flour to produce lighter, more easily digested breads and pastas. Spelt flour is often easier to tolerate than modern wheat because it is an unrefined grain type containing less gluten. You can also try gluten-free flour blends and buckwheat, chickpea and rice flours when baking. Note that agricultural spray residues may remain in the outer shells of intensively farmed grains, so choose organic.

Yeast: There are many types of yeast available. I use fresh yeast, but if you have another kind, just follow the instructions on the package.

To peel or not to peel: In the majority of vegetables, the highest concentration of micronutrients is found just under the skin, so I generally opt for non-peeling, even when making mashed potatoes (especially as the glycaemic index of vegetables rises when peeled). This ia another reason to buy organic. In most recipes I have not prescribed whether to peel, as you know the state of your vegetables and the preference of your dinner guests better than I do.

Preparing fruit: Always choose ripe fruit unless otherwise stated. Always rinse and prepare berries and fruit carefully before use.

NOTE
- The nutritional and calorie information for each recipe applies only to the ingredients listed (based on the first ingredient listed if alternatives are given), and not to any alternative options or additional serving suggestions (in *italic*).

BREAKFASTS

Berry Muesli

Starting the day with muesli, nuts, berries and yogurt is a sure-fire recipe for health. Packed with energy, vitamins, minerals, omega oils, antioxidants and other health-giving phytochemicals, nut and berry muesli has been proven to give beneficial effects to all body systems. It is also wonderfully quick to make and you can vary the berry combinations to suit the seasons and your changing needs.

Preparation time: 5 minutes | Calories per portion: 349

Serves 1

3 tbsp soy yogurt

50g/1¾oz/½ cup sugar-free muesli base

1 tbsp chopped nuts and seeds (such as walnuts, Brazil nuts, hazelnuts, sunflower seeds)

1 tbsp dried goji berries

1 tbsp desiccated/dried shredded coconut

3 tbsp fresh or frozen berries (see combinations below)

Put the yogurt in a bowl. Add the muesli, nuts, seeds and dried berries. Sprinkle the coconut and fresh berries on top. Serve with a glass of freshly squeezed grapefruit or orange juice, or a fresh fruit smoothie (see pages 200–209).

Tip: Using live yogurt (not long-life) helps to maintain a balanced intestinal flora for calm digestion and efficient nutrient absorption.

BERRY HEALTH-BOOSTER COMBINATIONS

For healthy joints
Elderberries, blackberries, cherries, loganberries, raspberries, strawberries

For the heart and circulation
Blueberries, blackcurrants, cherries, grapes, raspberries, strawberries

To avoid colds and infections
Cranberries, blackcurrants, kiwi fruit, gooseberries, redcurrants, elderberries

For healthy digestion
Blueberries, kiwi fruit, gooseberries, grapes, redcurrants

For healthy nerves and to improve memory
Blueberries, blackcurrants, gooseberries, raspberries

For healthy skin
Blueberries, cranberries, strawberries, kiwi fruit

Anti-cancer
Cherries, grapes, raspberries, strawberries

Detox
Grapes, loganberries, strawberries

NUTRITION PROFILE (per portion)
13% protein, 17% fat, 66% carbohydrate, 4% fibre

VITAMINS AND MINERALS (percentage of RDA)
Vitamin A 19%, E 73%, C 11%, B1 62%, B2 68%, B3 55%, B5 60%, B6 66%, folate 21%, potassium 29%, calcium 20%, phosphorus 42%, magnesium 21%, iron 47%, zinc 31%, copper 33%, manganese 111%, selenium 24%

HEALTH BENEFITS
Antioxidant | energy booster | immune stimulant | detox | digestive aid | helps lower cholesterol | reduces risk of heart disease

Açai Berry Breakfast Bowl

Raw oats make an ideal breakfast cereal. Known to help lower blood cholesterol and reduce the risk of heart disease, they are rich in dietary fibre and contain phytic acid, which may protect against cancer.

Preparation time: 5 minutes | Calories per portion: 341

Serves 1

1 banana, peeled and sliced

4 strawberries, hulled and sliced

1 tbsp açai berry pulp

3 tbsp soy yogurt

50g/1¾oz/½ cup rolled oats

1 tbsp chopped walnuts

1 tbsp chopped almonds

1 tbsp raisins

a pinch of ground cinnamon

Reserve a few slices of banana and strawberry to decorate the dish, then blend the remaining banana and strawberries, açai berry pulp and yogurt until smooth.

Place the oats, chopped walnuts and almonds (keeping a few to use as decoration) and raisins in a breakfast bowl. Sprinkle with cinnamon and add the açai fruit blend. Top with the reserved banana and strawberry slices and a scattering of chopped nuts.

Tip: To make a granola topping, mix the oats and nuts together with a little honey or maple syrup and roast them in the oven at 150°C/300°F/Gas 2 for about 10 minutes, or until just golden.

NUTRITION PROFILE (per portion)
11% protein, 29% fat, 55% carbohydrate, 5% fibre

VITAMINS AND MINERALS (percentage of RDA)
Vitamin E 15%, C 46%, B1 27%, B2 10%, B3 8%, B5 15%, B6 23%, folate 20%, biotin 11%, potassium 30%, calcium 8%, magnesium 27%, iron 19%, zinc 16%

HEALTH BENEFITS
Lowers blood sugar and cholesterol levels | may improve mental function | reduces oxidative stress | reduces risk of heart disease | anti-cancer

Raw-Food Breakfast

Sprouted seeds are among the most nutritious foods available as the sprouting process increases the concentration of vital nutrients and makes the seeds easier to digest.

Preparation time: 10 minutes, plus soaking and sprouting | Calories per portion: 324

Serves 4

200g/7oz/1 cup whole (unhulled) oats, soaked and sprouted (see below)

50g/1¾oz/⅓ cup sunflower seeds, soaked and sprouted (see below)

100g/3½oz cherries, halved and pitted

2 thick slices of watermelon, peeled, deseeded and cubed

1 papaya, peeled, deseeded and cubed

2 bananas, peeled and sliced

4 kiwi fruit, peeled and sliced

50g/1¾oz/heaped ⅓ cup Brazil nuts, chopped

juice from 1 orange

Rinse and cover the oats and sunflower seeds with water and soak for approximately 8 hours. Change the water and soak again for another 8 hours. Drain off the water, then place the oats and seeds in a wide-necked jar, covered with a piece of muslin/cheesecloth or mesh, and leave to sprout for 24 hours, or until you can see little shoots. Drain off any residual water and rinse the sprouted seeds before using.

Mix all the fruits and nuts together with the sprouted seeds in a large bowl and serve.

NUTRITION PROFILE (per portion)
11% protein, 35% fat, 49% carbohydrate, 5% fibre

VITAMINS AND MINERALS (percentage of RDA)
Vitamin E 41%, C 72%, B1 56%, B2 10%, B3 9%, B5 17%, B6 23%, folate 20%, biotin 10%, potassium 40%, calcium 12%, phosphorus 56%, magnesium 55%, iron 26%, zinc 29%, copper 85%, manganese 135%, selenium 59%

HEALTH BENEFITS
Antioxidant | immune booster | benefits hair and skin | good for cholesterol, heart, blood and circulation | improves sleep and mood | aids digestion

Sweet Oat Porridge

Preparation and cooking time: 10 minutes | Calories per portion: 382

Serves 1

3–4 tbsp rolled oats

1 tsp chopped hazelnuts

1 tbsp dried berries (goji, cranberries, blueberries, raisins)

soy milk, to taste

To serve

3 tbsp berries, fresh or frozen

1 tsp clear honey

Put the oats in a saucepan with the nuts and dried berries. Add about twice the volume of water and bring to the boil, stirring continuously. Simmer gently for a few minutes until the porridge/oatmeal thickens. Gradually add a little milk for a rich, creamy consistency. Serve topped with the fresh or frozen berries and a drizzle of honey.

NUTRITION PROFILE (per portion)

13% protein, 30% fat, 50% carbohydrate, 7% fibre

VITAMINS AND MINERALS (percentage of RDA)

Vitamin E 31%, C 49%, B1 49%, B2 31%, B3 10%, B5 22%, B6 21%, folate 47%, biotin 21%, potassium 33%, calcium 12%, phosphorus 56%, magnesium 39%, iron 32%, zinc 31%, copper 64%, manganese 195%

HEALTH BENEFITS

Antioxidant | immune booster | helps prevent infections | provides steady energy and brain food | helps prevent cystitis and prostate problems | improves circulation

Raw Cloudberry Compôte and Yogurt

One of the easiest breakfasts to whip up, this also doubles as a healthy snack. Cloudberry compôte is a beautiful golden-coloured sauce that can also form the basis of a delicious dessert when served with ice cream or cake.

Preparation time: 5 minutes | Calories per portion: 230

Serves 2

200g/7oz cloudberries

2 tbsp maple syrup

400ml/14fl oz/1⅔ cups plain soy yogurt

ground cinnamon (optional)

Blend the cloudberries with the maple syrup until smooth, then serve as a topping over the yogurt, with a sprinkling of cinnamon for added spice, if you like. Serve immediately, or cover and keep in the refrigerator for up to 3 days.

Tip: Substitute the cloudberries to make a compote with raspberries, boysenberries, dewberries, loganberries, mulberries or blackberries.

NUTRITION PROFILE (per portion)

22% protein, 34% fat, 38% carbohydrate, 6% fibre

VITAMINS AND MINERALS (percentage of RDA)

Vitamin A 6%, E 29%, C 40%, folate 16%, calcium 5%, magnesium 6%, iron 8%, zinc 9%, copper 11%, manganese 46%

HEALTH BENEFITS

Antioxidant | boosts immunity | improves digestion

Scotch Pancakes with Berries and Jujube Syrup

Scotch pancakes, also commonly known as drop scones, are a simple and easy dessert that children enjoy helping make. Jujube syrup has a rich, sweet, date-like flavour that goes particularly well with these light, fluffy pancakes.

Preparation and cooking time: 1 hour | Calories per portion: 233

Serves 4

For the jujube syrup

100g/3½oz dried jujube berries

50g/1¾oz/¼ cup raw cane sugar

For the Scotch pancakes

125g/4½oz/1 cup plain/all-pupose flour

1 tsp baking powder

1 tbsp sugar

50g/1¾oz vegetable margarine, diced

1 egg, beaten

150ml/5fl oz/⅔ cup soy milk

grapeseed, corn or coconut oil, for frying

To serve

250g/9oz/1 cup ice cream

100g/3½oz fresh raspberries or strawberries

100g/3½oz honeyberries (optional)

Place the jujube berries in a saucepan with 200ml/7fl oz/scant 1 cup water and half the sugar. Bring to the boil, then turn the heat down to low and simmer gently, partially covered, for 20 minutes. Stir in the rest of the sugar, bring back to the boil and then simmer again for about 20 minutes until you have a glossy syrup with sweet rehydrated jujube berries. Use immediately or cool, cover and store in the refrigerator for 2–3 days.

For the Scotch pancakes, sift the flour and baking powder into a bowl. Mix in the sugar, then add the margarine by chopping it into the flour with a knife and spoon until it forms small lumps. Crumble the dough with your fingers until the mixture resembles fine breadcrumbs, then mix in the egg. Stir in the milk, a little at a time, to make a smooth, thick batter.

Heat a little oil in a large frying pan over a medium-low heat. Use a tablespoon to pour the batter into the hot pan to make small round pancakes with enough space around them to be able to turn them easily. Cook for about 1–2 minutes on each side until golden. Keep the pancakes warm covered in a clean dish towel, or serve as you go.

Serve the pancakes warm with a dollop of ice cream, the jujube syrup, a few fresh berries and the honeyberries scattered on top, if you like.

Tip: Jujube berries are also called 'Chinese dates' and can be found in Asian grocers and supermarkets. For a vegan option, you can use a natural egg replacer, such as No Egg, or 1 teaspoon extra of baking powder.

NUTRITION PROFILE (per portion)
10% protein, 39% fat, 48% carbohydrate, 3% fibre

VITAMINS AND MINERALS (percentage of RDA)
Vitamin A 14%, D 19%, E 5%, C 8%, B1 13%, B2 17% B3 7%, B5 8%, B6 9%, B12 13%, folate 12%, biotin 6%, potassium 13%, calcium 10%, magnesium 10%, iron 10%

HEALTH BENEFITS
Soothing and satisfying | provides a source of quick energy

Breakfast Bagel

Preparation time: 5 minutes | Calories per portion: 378

Serves 1

2 tbsp cream cheese

1 bagel, split and toasted

3 slices of tomato

1 tsp capers, rinsed

Spread the cream cheese onto the toasted bagel halves. Add the tomatoes and capers and serve immediately.

Tip: As a sweet variation, try topping the cream cheese with blueberries and sliced strawberries, a little honey or syrup and some fresh mint. Use plant-based cream cheese for a vegan option.

NUTRITION PROFILE (per portion)
11% protein, 33% fat, 54% carbohydrate, 2% fibre

VITAMINS AND MINERALS (percentage of RDA)
Vitamin A 25%, E 13%, C 22%, B1 9%, B3 7%, B5 5%, B6 11%, folate 14%, potassium 15%, magnesium 7%, iron 5%

HEALTH BENEFITS
Nourishing | antioxidant | improves eyesight and skin | strengthens muscles

French Toast with Rose Hip Coulis

Preparation and cooking time: 20 minutes | Calories per portion: 354

Serves 4

For the rose hip coulis

200g/7oz rose hips, trimmed, deseeded and rinsed (see page 153)

50g/1¾oz/¼ cup raw cane sugar

For the French toast

4 eggs

100ml/3½fl oz/scant ½ cup soy milk

2 tsp ground cinnamon

8 thick slices of French country bread
(preferably slightly stale)

olive oil, for frying

Put the rose hips and sugar in a saucepan with 100ml/3½fl oz/scant ½ cup water and bring to the boil, then reduce the heat, cover and leave to simmer gently for about 10 minutes, or until the rose hips are soft. Blend the mixture to a smooth purée and leave to cool while you make the French toast.

Beat the eggs, milk and cinnamon together in a shallow dish. Dip each slice of bread in the egg mixture for a few seconds until the liquid is soaked up. Heat the oil in a large frying pan and fry the soaked bread in batches until golden brown on both sides. Serve with the coulis.

NUTRITION PROFILE (per portion)
16% protein, 39% fat, 42% carbohydrate, 3% fibre

VITAMINS AND MINERALS (percentage of RDA)
Vitamin A 13%, D 18%, E 9%, C 74%, B1 22%, B2 26%, B3 15%, B5 21%, B6 15%, B12 50%, folate 33%, biotin 25%, potassium 14%, calcium 25%, phosphorus 34%, magnesium 12%, iron 24%, zinc 18%, copper 20%, selenium 15%, iodine 21%

HEALTH BENEFITS
Antioxidant | good immune and energy booster | good for skin, bones, mucous membranes, hair and nails

Hash Browns with Sweet Chilli, Tomato and Goji Berry Sauce

These are good served as they are or, for a more substantial breakfast, select a combination from the following: baked beans, grilled/broiled sausages and tomatoes, scrambled eggs or tofu, fried mushrooms and plenty of toast.

Preparation and cooking time: 40 minutes | Calories per portion: 260

Serves 4

For the hash browns

2 large baking potatoes, scrubbed and
 roughly cubed
1 small onion, finely chopped
1 garlic clove, crushed
olive oil, for frying
sea salt and freshly ground black pepper

For the sweet chilli, tomato and goji berry sauce

100g/3½oz red chillies, deseeded
1 garlic clove
100g/3½oz tomatoes, quartered
3 tbsp dried goji berries
3 tbsp red wine vinegar
125g/4½oz/⅔ cup raw cane sugar

Put the potatoes in a pan of salted water. Bring to the boil, then turn the heat down and simmer for about 15 minutes until tender.

Meanwhile, prepare the sauce. Blend the chillies, garlic and tomatoes until finely chopped. Transfer the purée to a saucepan and add the goji berries, vinegar and sugar. Heat slowly over a medium heat until the sugar dissolves, stirring occasionally. Bring to the boil, then reduce the heat and simmer, stirring now and again, for about 15 minutes until the sauce thickens.

Drain the potatoes and mash roughly with the onion and garlic. Season with salt and pepper, then shape into 4 flat patties.

Heat a little oil in a frying pan and cook the patties over a medium heat until they are brown on both sides. Take care not to use too much oil or the hash browns will disintegrate. Serve with the sauce.

NUTRITION PROFILE (per portion)
9% protein, 10% fat, 78% carbohydrate, 3% fibre

VITAMINS AND MINERALS (percentage of RDA)
Vitamin A 24%, C 90%, B1 25%, B6 28%, potassium 26%, calcium 15%, magnesium 7%, iron 23%, copper 15%

HEALTH BENEFITS
Antioxidant | gives steady energy | immune booster | improves blood and circulation | aids liver function | improves cell respiration | lowers cholesterol

LIGHT MEALS

Carrot and Goji Berry Soup

Preparation and cooking time: 30 minutes | Calories per portion: 141

Serves 4

1kg/2lb 4oz carrots, thinly sliced

100g/3½oz dried goji berries

2.5cm/1in piece of root ginger, finely chopped

1l/35fl oz/4¼ cups vegetable stock

500ml/17fl oz/2 cups orange juice

1 bunch of coriander/cilantro leaves, finely chopped, plus extra leaves to serve

sea salt and freshly ground black pepper

Place the carrots, goji berries and ginger in a large saucepan with the stock and the orange juice. Bring quickly to the boil over a high heat, then reduce the heat and simmer, covered, for 15 minutes, or until the carrots are soft. Blend to a smooth, creamy consistency.

Stir in the chopped coriander/cilantro leaves and add salt and pepper to taste. Sprinkle with extra coriander/cilantro leaves and serve hot or cold.

NUTRITION PROFILE (per portion)

11% protein, 6% fat, 73% carbohydrate, 10% fibre

VITAMINS AND MINERALS (percentage of RDA)

Vitamin A 471%, E 9%, C 81%, B1 27%, B2 4%, B3%, B5 10%, B6 22%, folate 25%, potassium 27%, calcium 11%, magnesium 5%, iron 17%, zinc 3%, selenium 3%

HEALTH BENEFITS

Low calorie | high in vitamin A and antioxidants | good for eyes and skin | protects against infections, cancer and heart disease

Wild Rice and Strawberry Salad

Preparation and cooking time: 50 minutes | Calories per portion: 219

Serves 4

100g/3½oz/½ cup wild rice

2 tbsp walnut oil

4 tbsp Raspberry Vinegar (see page 187)

25g/1oz hazelnuts, finely chopped

25g/1oz almonds, finely chopped

2 spring onions/scallions, finely chopped

500g/1lb 2oz strawberries, hulled and sliced

sea salt

Put the rice in a pan of cold salted water. Cook according to the package instructions until all the water is absorbed. Leave to cool and then mix in the walnut oil and the raspberry vinegar.

Toast the nuts in a dry frying pan with a little salt until just golden.

Place the rice in a large salad bowl. Add the toasted nuts, spring onions/scallions and strawberries. Toss together gently and serve.

NUTRITION PROFILE (per portion)

11% protein, 48% fat, 36% carbohydrate, 5% fibre

VITAMINS AND MINERALS (percentage of RDA)

Vitamin E 22%, C 94%, B1 8%, B2 9%, B3 13%, B5 10%, B6 13%, folate 24%, biotin 15%, potassium 17%, magnesium 17%, iron 9%, zinc 15%, copper 28%, iodine 6%

HEALTH BENEFITS

Benefits cell membranes, skin, hair and nails | helps protect against infection and degenerative disorders | encourages stable blood sugar level

Roast Butternut Squash and Redcurrant Salad

Preparation and cooking time: 40 minutes | Calories per portion: 187

Serves 4

1 butternut squash, peeled, deseeded and cubed

3 garlic cloves, crushed

4 oregano sprigs, leaves chopped

2 tbsp olive oil

2 courgettes/zucchini, halved lengthways and sliced

25g/1oz pine nuts

100g/3½oz rocket/arugula

100g/3½oz redcurrants, rinsed and stalks removed

2 tbsp balsamic vinegar

sea salt and freshly ground black pepper

Preheat the oven to 200°C/400°F/Gas 6. Place the butternut squash in a roasting pan. Sprinkle with the garlic and season with salt, plenty of pepper and half the oregano. Drizzle with 1 tablespoon of the oil and roast in the oven for 20 minutes.

Meanwhile, stir-fry the courgettes/zucchini and pine nuts in the remaining oil until they start to brown. Season with salt and pepper, and sprinkle with the remaining oregano.

Put the rocket/arugula in a large shallow bowl. Place the butternut squash, courgettes/zucchini and pine nuts on top. Sprinkle with the redcurrants and balsamic vinegar and serve.

NUTRITION PROFILE (per portion)
10% protein, 57% fat, 28% carbohydrate, 5% fibre

VITAMINS AND MINERALS (percentage of RDA)
Vitamin A 95%, E 29%, C 57%, B1 20%, B3 8%, B5 10%, B6 19%, folate 35%, potassium 39%, calcium 18%, phosphorus 18%, magnesium 23%, iron 16%, zinc 10%, copper 23%, manganese 44%

HEALTH BENEFITS
Anti-cancer | good for heart and blood cells | benefits skin, muscles and nerves

Waldorf Salad

Preparation time: 10 minutes, plus 30 minutes chilling | Calories per portion: 175

Serves 4

100ml/3½fl oz/scant ½ cup crème fraîche
 or plant-based whipping cream
1 tbsp raw cane sugar
250g/9oz seedless red grapes, halved
200g/7oz celeriac, grated

2 celery stalks, finely sliced, leaves reserved
 for sprinkling
2 red apples, cored and cubed
50g/1¾oz/⅓ cup walnuts, chopped
sea salt
lettuce, to serve

Mix the crème fraîche with the sugar and a pinch of salt in a bowl. Fold in the rest of the ingredients, reserving a few grapes and walnuts for serving. Refrigerate, covered, for at least 30 minutes. Serve on a bed of lettuce, sprinkled with the reserved grapes, celery leaves and walnuts.

NUTRITION PROFILE (per portion)
6% protein, 60% fat, 31% carbohydrate, 3% fibre

VITAMINS AND MINERALS (percentage of RDA)
Vitamin A 12%, E 6%, C 10%, B1 13%, B6 10%, folate 16%, potassium 18%, calcium 5%, magnesium 7%, iron 6%

HEALTH BENEFITS
Antioxidant and anti-inflammatory | helps lower blood cholesterol and prevents blood clot formation

Spinach, Tomato and Persimmon Salad

Preparation time: 10 minutes | Calories per portion: 211

Serves 4

200g/7oz young spinach leaves, rinsed
and drained

2 beefsteak tomatoes, thinly sliced

200g/7oz cherry tomatoes, halved

2 persimmons, thinly sliced

½ red onion, thinly sliced

6 Brazil nuts, chopped

extra virgin olive oil, for drizzling

balsamic vinegar, for drizzling

sea salt and freshly ground black pepper

Spread the spinach on a shallow serving dish. Add the tomatoes, persimmons and red onion and top with the Brazil nuts. Drizzle with the oil and vinegar, toss, season to taste and serve.

NUTRITION PROFILE (per portion)
12% protein, 33% fat, 46% carbohydrate, 9% fibre

VITAMINS AND MINERALS (percentage of RDA)
Vitamin A 84%, E 21%, C 40%, B1 16%, B2 4%, B3 10%, B5 7%, B6 20%, folate 37%, biotin 4%, potassium 29%, calcium 11%, magnesium 13%, iron 11%, copper 15%, manganese 28%, selenium 20%, iodine 3%

HEALTH BENEFITS
Low calorie but boosts energy levels | benefits blood and microcirculation | helps fight infections and cell deterioration

Smoked Trout, Quinoa and Grape Salad

Preparation and cooking time: 20 minutes, plus 15 minutes soaking | Calories per portion: 329

Serves 4

150g/5½oz/scant 1 cup quinoa

100g/3½oz seedless red grapes, halved

100g/3½oz celeriac, cut into small cubes

50g/1¾oz/⅓ cup walnuts, chopped

1 red apple, cored and cut into thin slices

1 tbsp mayonnaise

2 tsp coarse mustard

crisp lettuce leaves

4 smoked trout fillets, skin and bones
    removed, or 250g/9oz smoked tofu, sliced

2 tsp chopped dill, for sprinkling

sea salt and freshly ground black pepper

Put the quinoa in a pan and soak in cold water for 15 minutes. Drain and rinse several times. After the last rinse, add 250ml/9fl oz/1 cup cold water and a pinch of salt to the pan. Bring to the boil, cover and simmer for 15 minutes, adding more water if necessary. Remove from the heat and let stand for 5 minutes with the lid on.

Meanwhile, mix the grapes, celeriac, walnuts and apple in a bowl with the mayonnaise and mustard. Leave to chill in the refrigerator for at least 10 minutes.

Make a bed of lettuce and set the trout on top. Fluff the quinoa gently with a fork and serve with the grape salad. Season to taste and sprinkle over the dill.

NUTRITION PROFILE (per portion)
27% protein, 42% fat, 28% carbohydrate, 3% fibre

VITAMINS AND MINERALS (percentage of RDA)
Vitamin A 9%, D 166%, E 16%, C 9%, B1 34%, B2 18%, B3 30%, B5 25%, B6 28%, folate 29%, biotin 10%, potassium 44%, calcium 10%, magnesium 31%, iron 25%, zinc 19%, copper 46%, manganese 30%, selenium 28%, iodine 9%

HEALTH BENEFITS
High in omega oils | benefits bones, muscles, nerves and memory | helps strengthen heart and circulation

Shawarma with Golden Berry Chutney

A *shawarma* is a Middle Eastern meat wrap or pitta sandwich made with thinly sliced, spiced meat. For a vegan version, substitute seitan for the chicken.

Preparation and cooking time: 30 minutes, plus 1 hour marinating | Calories per portion: 256

Serves 4

For the shawarma

400g/14oz boneless, skinless chicken breast fillet or seitan, sliced thinly

3–4 garlic cloves, crushed

1 tsp sea salt

1 tsp freshly ground black pepper

1 tsp ground allspice

1 tsp ground cardamom

½ tsp ground mace

200ml/7fl oz/scant 1 cup soy yogurt

1 persimmon, finely chopped

3 tbsp lemon juice

For the golden berry chutney

100g/3½oz fresh or 50g/1¾oz dried golden berries

1 persimmon, finely chopped

1 small red onion, finely chopped

1 red chilli, finely chopped

1 handful of coriander/cilantro leaves, finely chopped

1 tbsp olive oil

4 pitta bread, warmed, to serve

Mix all the shawarma ingredients together in a bowl, cover and leave to marinate in the refrigerator for at least 1 hour (or overnight). Meanwhile, blend all the chutney ingredients to make a coarse paste.

Drain off the marinade, then grill/broil or fry the chicken slices for 5–8 minutes, turning occasionally until cooked through and golden. Serve in the warmed pitta breads with the chutney.

Tip: Mango makes a good substitute for persimmon in the chutney.

To make a more substantial dish, serve with Açai-Tahini Sauce (see page 144), hummus, lettuce, cucumber, red onion and tomato slices, as well as the golden berry chutney.

NUTRITION PROFILE (per portion)
37% protein, 37% fat, 23% carbohydrate, 3% fibre

VITAMINS AND MINERALS (percentage of RDA)
Vitamin A 10%, E 10%, C 43%, B1 28%, B2 13%, B3 47%, B5 20%, B6 33%, biotin 5%, potassium 30%, calcium 9%, magnesium 18%, iron 26%, zinc 17%, copper 25%, manganese 33%, selenium 33%

HEALTH BENEFITS
High protein | filling yet low calorie | antioxidant | enables healing | strengthens bones, teeth and mucous membranes | anti-inflammatory | improves metabolism | helps stress relief

Salmon with Tapenade

You can substitute the salmon in this dish with tofu for a vegan alternative. This is good served with hot toast and a green salad.

Preparation and cooking time: 20 minutes | Calories per portion: 255

Serves 4

4 salmon fillets, or 450g/1lb firm tofu, sliced

lemon juice

sea salt

For the tapenade

100g/3½oz drained caperberries

100g/3½oz black olives, pitted

1 red pepper, deseeded

1 bunch of parsley leaves

1 bunch of mint leaves

1 tbsp extra virgin olive oil

Prepare the salmon by scraping the scales off the skin with a sharp knife. Turn the fillets over and rub the other sides with salt and lemon juice. Grill/broil the fillets skin-side up for 5–6 minutes until crisp and golden. Turn over and cook for 1 minute.

Meanwhile, make the tapenade by blending all the ingredients to make a coarse paste. Serve immediately with the salmon, or keep covered in the refrigerator for up to 3 days, but return to room temperature before serving.

NUTRITION PROFILE (per portion)
33% protein, 60% fat, 5% carbohydrate, 2% fibre

VITAMINS AND MINERALS (percentage of RDA)
Vitamin A 31%, D 112%, E 29%, C 74%, B1 24%, B2 14%, B3 47%, B5 17%, B6 59%, B12 151%, folate 27%, biotin 13%, potassium 26%, calcium 11%, magnesium 12%, iron 20%, copper 18%, manganese 11%, selenium 46%, iodine 24%

HEALTH BENEFITS
Nourishing | high in omega 3 and antioxidants | encourages calcium absorption | helps protect against infections

Woodland Roast Stuffed Mushrooms

Preparation and cooking time: 30 minutes | Calories per portion: 253

Serves 4

12 large open Portobello mushrooms

1 tbsp olive oil, plus extra for greasing

3 garlic cloves

50g/1¾oz/½ cup dry breadcrumbs

50g/1¾oz cream cheese

½ tsp harissa paste or finely chopped red chilli

1 tsp dried thyme

200g/7oz raspberries, blackberries and/or dewberries, rinsed

Preheat the oven to 200°C/400°F/Gas 6. Clean the mushrooms, snap off the stalks at the base and reserve. Place the caps upside down in a greased ovenproof dish. Finely chop the mushroom stalks and the garlic together. Heat the oil in a sauté pan, add the chopped stalks and garlic and stir-fry for 2 minutes, or until the mushroom stalks give off their liquid. Add the breadcrumbs and stir until they have soaked up all the liquid. Remove from the heat and leave to cool for a few minutes, then stir in the cream cheese, harissa paste, thyme and fresh berries. Fill the mushroom caps with the stem and berry mixture, pressing it down well. Bake for 10–15 minutes until golden. Serve immediately.

Serve with steamed green beans, creamed spinach and rice.

NUTRITION PROFILE (per portion)
17% protein, 40% fat, 38% carbohydrate, 5% fibre

VITAMINS AND MINERALS (percentage of RDA)
Vitamin A 19%, D 1%, E 9%, C 54%, B1 20%, B2 35%, B3 33%, B5 48%, B6 26%, B12 2%, folate 45%, biotin 34%, potassium 35%, calcium 11%, magnesium 24%, iron 24%, zinc 11%, copper 110%, manganese 42%, selenium 23%, iodine 3%

HEALTH BENEFITS
Low calorie | high energy release | helps keep blood cells healthy | protects against inflammation, osteoporosis and arthritis

Lentil, Tomato and Aronia Flan

Make the pastry dough before you start to prepare the lentil filling so that it has time to chill in the refrigerator before being rolled out.

Preparation and cooking time: 1 hour | Calories per portion: 426

Serves 4

For the pastry dough

250g/9oz/scant 2 cups plain/all-purpose flour

½ tsp sea salt

125g/4½oz cold vegetable margarine, diced, plus extra for greasing

For the filling

125g/4½oz/⅔ cup dried red lentils, rinsed

1 tbsp olive oil

3 shallots, chopped

½ tsp turmeric

a pinch of cayenne pepper

1 yellow pepper, deseeded and sliced

2 tbsp tomato purée/paste

1 tbsp sugar

150g/5½oz aronia berries

8 cherry tomatoes, sliced

sea salt and freshly ground black pepper

Mix the flour and salt in a bowl. Add the margarine by chopping it into the flour with a knife and spoon until it forms small lumps. Continue to rub the fat into the flour with your fingers until the mixture resembles fine breadcrumbs. Gradually add about 70ml/2¼fl oz/¼ cup cold water to make a soft dough. Roll into a ball, wrap in cling film/plastic wrap and leave to chill in the refrigerator while you make the filling.

Preheat the oven to 200°C/400°F/Gas 6 and grease a 22cm/8½in round baking pan. Put the lentils into a saucepan, cover with water and bring to the boil. Turn the heat down to low and leave to simmer for about 15 minutes. In another saucepan, gently heat the oil and sauté the shallots for 2 minutes over a medium-high heat. Add the spices, then the yellow pepper and heat through. Using a slotted spoon, add the lentils, then pour over enough of their cooking liquid to cover. Bring to the boil, then turn the heat down and add the tomato purée/paste, sugar and aronia berries. Leave to simmer gently while you roll out the dough to fit the prepared pan. Gently press the dough into the pan.

Season the filling to taste with salt and pepper. Transfer to the pastry case/pie shell, smooth the top and decorate with the cherry tomato slices. Bake in the middle of the oven for 25–30 minutes until golden, then serve.

Serve with a green salad or steamed green vegetables.

Tip: You can use whole blackcurrants or blueberries instead of aronia berries.

NUTRITION PROFILE (per portion)
13% protein, 35% fat, 47% carbohydrate, 5% fibre

VITAMINS AND MINERALS (percentage of RDA)
Vitamin A 34%, E 25%, C 53%, B1 35%, B2 10%, B3 25%, B5 14%, B6 39%, folate 29%, biotin 8%, potassium 31%, calcium 7%, magnesium 34%, iron 34%, zinc 25%, copper 42%, manganese 81%, selenium 9%, iodine 1%

HEALTH BENEFITS
Boosts metabolism | protects heart and circulation | helps lower cholesterol | can help relieve problems associated with diabetes

SNACKS AND
SIDE DISHES

Berry Trail Mix

A combination of berries, nuts and chocolate makes the perfect snack for hikers or people on the go.

Preparation time: 3 minutes | Calories per portion: 121

Serves 4

1 tbsp dried cranberries

1 tbsp dried goji berries

1 tbsp dried blueberries

1 tbsp raisins

1 tbsp dried rose hips

2 tbsp peanuts

2 tbsp Brazil nuts, roughly chopped

2 tbsp cashew nuts

2 tbsp almonds

2 tbsp walnuts, roughly chopped

2 tbsp dark/bittersweet chocolate chips

Mix all the ingredients together in a bowl. Put in small sandwich bags and take as a snack on hikes and outings. Store in an airtight container if not using immediately.

NUTRITION PROFILE (per portion)
11% protein, 52% fat, 32% carbohydrate, 5% fibre

VITAMINS AND MINERALS (percentage of RDA)
Vitamin E 10%, C 30%, B1 8%, potassium 9%, calcium 5%, magnesium 9%, zinc 5%, copper 18%, manganese 15%, selenium 12%

HEALTH BENEFITS
Gives steady energy | repairs tissue and improves cell respiration

Tomato Crisps

Try these with savoury dips such as hummus, tapenade and tzatziki.

Preparation and cooking time: 35 minutes | Calories per portion: 77

Serves 4

5 beefsteak tomatoes, quartered and deseeded

2 tsp sugar

1 tsp sea salt

2 tsp potato flour

2 tsp herbes de Provence

Preheat the oven to 100°C/200°F/Gas ½. Blend all the ingredients to a smooth consistency. Spread the tomato mixture thinly onto a baking sheet lined with baking parchment and bake for about 30 minutes until crisp and completely dry.

Break into chips and serve with dips or salsa.

Tip: Tomato crisps can also be made successfully in a dehydrator.

NUTRITION PROFILE (per portion)
12% protein, 10% fat, 71% carbohydrate, 7% fibre

VITAMINS AND MINERALS (percentage of RDA)
Vitamin A 26%, E 19%, C 42%, B1 15%, B3 13%, B5 9%, B6 19%, folate 21%, biotin 6%, potassium 32%, calcium 9%, magnesium 20%, iron 20%, manganese 23%

HEALTH BENEFITS
Anti-cancer | good for muscles, skin, eyes and bones | benefits blood sugar and cholesterol | helps immunity and stress relief

Chocolate-Dipped Strawberries

Preparation and cooking time: 10 minutes, plus setting | Calories per portion: 159

Serves 4

250g/9oz whole strawberries

100g/3½oz/⅔ cup dark/bittersweet chocolate chips

2 tbsp chopped almonds

Rinse the strawberries and rest on paper towels to dry.

Heat the chocolate in a glass bowl over a pan of simmering water until just melted. Remove from the heat and stir until smooth.

Meanwhile, toast the almonds in a frying pan until they start to turn golden, then transfer to a bowl.

Hold the strawberries by the stem end and dip them one by one, first in the chocolate, then in the chopped almonds. Leave to set on baking parchment for about 30 minutes, then serve.

NUTRITION PROFILE (per portion)
6% protein, 55% fat, 37% carbohydrate, 2% fibre

VITAMINS AND MINERALS (percentage of RDA)
Vitamin E 11%, C 48%, biotin 8%

HEALTH BENEFITS
Invigorating snack for children | antioxidant | anti-inflammatory | anti-cancer | good for eyes, bones and nails | may improve circulation and blood sugar control

Avocado and Kiwi Appetizer

This is best served with some toasted bread.

Preparation time: 10 minutes | Calories per portion: 129

Serves 4

1 tsp Dijon mustard

1cm/½in piece of root ginger, grated

1 tbsp olive oil

1 tbsp white wine vinegar

1 lettuce, shredded

2 avocados, peeled, pitted and sliced

4 kiwi fruit, peeled and sliced

sea salt and freshly ground black pepper

Put the mustard in a small bowl. Stir in the ginger and season with salt and pepper, then add the oil very slowly, stirring all the time. Slowly add the vinegar, stirring continuously. Add a little warm water, if necessary, to achieve a smooth consistency. Adjust the seasoning to taste.

Toss the lettuce with 2 tablespoons of the dressing, then arrange a small bed of lettuce onto four plates. Place the avocado and kiwi slices on top and drizzle with the remaining dressing.

NUTRITION PROFILE (per portion)
6% protein, 68% fat, 20% carbohydrate, 6% fibre

VITAMINS AND MINERALS (percentage of RDA)
Vitamin A 15%, E 13%, C 38%, B1 11%, B2 6%, B3 5%, B5 8%, B6 15%, folate 20%, potassium 21%, calcium 5%, magnesium 5%, iron 6%

HEALTH BENEFITS
Low calorie | high in unsaturated fats | good for heart, circulation and skin | promotes healthy bones and joints | encourages tissue repair

Greek Caperberry Pâté

Preparation time: 5 minutes | Calories per portion: 156

Serves 4

200g/7oz/1 cup cooked butter/lima beans

50g/1¾oz/⅓ cup macadamia nuts

100g/3½oz drained caperberries

2 tbsp olive oil

1 small green chilli, deseeded

sea salt

Place all the ingredients in a bowl and blend or mash together until smooth. Store in the refrigerator in an airtight container, but return to room temperature before serving.

Serve with oatcakes/crackers or toast and a tomato salad.

Tip: For added colour and texture, serve with slices of lime, radishes, red pepper and tomatoes.

NUTRITION PROFILE (per portion)
9% protein, 68% fat, 14% carbohydrate, 9% fibre

VITAMINS AND MINERALS (percentage of RDA)
Vitamin C 13%, E 8%, B1 23%, B6 7%, potassium 9%, calcium 6%, magnesium 11%, iron 11%, zinc 6%, copper 23%, manganese 42%

HEALTH BENEFITS
Light but filling | good for digestion | benefits blood, veins and capillaries

Red Grape Rolls

Preparation time: 15 minutes | Calories per portion: 128

Serves 4

1 spring onion/scallion, finely sliced

16 seedless red grapes, halved or quartered

1 avocado, peeled, pitted and diced

1 carrot, grated

1cm/½in slice of celeriac, grated

8 walnut halves, chopped

1 handful of bean sprouts

8 large lettuce leaves

Mix together all the ingredients, except the lettuce leaves, in a bowl. Place a small handful of the mixture in each lettuce leaf. Roll each leaf into a cone shape and secure with a cocktail stick/toothpick.

These are good served with hummus, tzatziki sauce, tahini or French dressing as a dipping accompaniment.

NUTRITION PROFILE (per portion)
8% protein, 67% fat, 20% carbohydrate, 5% fibre

VITAMINS AND MINERALS (percentage of RDA)
Vitamin A 26%, E 11%, C 10%, B1 13%, B5 9%, B6 15%, folate 22%, potassium 19%, calcium 4%, magnesium 7%, iron 7%, zinc 5%, manganese 23%, copper 18%

HEALTH BENEFITS
Low calorie | quick energy release | antioxidant | benefits eyes, skin, muscles and joints | diuretic

Oyster Mushroom, Hijiki and Gooseberry Ramekins

Hijiki dried seaweed is sold in health food shops, Asian food stores and supermarkets.

Preparation and cooking time: 40 minutes | Calories per portion: 198

Serves 4

125g/4½oz ready-made puff pastry

15g/½oz/about ¾ cup dried hijiki

500g/1lb 2oz oyster mushrooms, cut into julienne strips

1 tbsp olive oil, plus extra for sautéing and greasing

1 tbsp chopped tarragon leaves

1 small bunch of chervil, ends trimmed

1 small carrot, cut into julienne strips

1 small leek, cut into julienne strips

200g/7oz gooseberries, trimmed

1 tbsp dry white wine

sea salt and freshly ground black pepper

Grease four 240ml/8fl oz/1 cup ramekins, each about 10cm/4in in diameter. Roll out the puff pastry dough into a 1cm/½in thick square. Use a ramekin dish as a template to cut out 4 lids, each one about 1cm/½in wider in diameter than the ramekin. Chill the dough lids in the refrigerator.

Soak the hijiki for 5 minutes in 500ml/17fl oz/2 cups cold water. Sauté the mushrooms in a little oil until golden, then leave to one side. Bring 100ml/3½fl oz/scant ½ cup water to the boil in a small saucepan with a pinch of salt, the oil, tarragon and chervil. Add the carrot, leek and drained hijiki and cook for 2 minutes. Add the gooseberries and cook for 1 more minute. Strain the liquid into another pan and leave the vegetables to cool. Add the wine to the liquid in the pan and boil for 2 minutes. Season to taste and leave to one side.

Preheat the oven to 220°C/425°F/Gas 7. Divide the vegetables and gooseberries evenly into four ramekins. Top with the mushrooms and a spoonful of the vegetable stock. Brush the ramekin edges with a little oil. Cover with the dough lids, pressing down firmly to keep them in place. Slit the lids in two or three places with a fork or a sharp knife. Bake for 10 minutes at the top of the hot oven until golden and serve.

Tip: Try using kiwi fruit instead of gooseberries. You can also experiment with other berries such as aronia, jujube, blueberries or red currants.

NUTRITION PROFILE (per portion)
11% protein, 44% fat, 38% carbohydrate, 7% fibre

VITAMINS AND MINERALS (percentage of RDA)
Vitamin A 17%, C 19%, B1 18%, B2 36%, B3 8%, B6 12%, folate 12%, potassium 22%, calcium 11%, magnesium 15%, iron 25%, selenium 16%, iodine 8%

HEALTH BENEFITS
Promotes healthy bones | aids protein and fat metabolism | maintains healthy cell membranes and supports tissue repair | benefits heart and joints

Cauliflower Juniper

Adding vinegar to the cauliflower cooking water brings out the flavour of the cauliflower and makes it easier to digest.

Preparation and cooking time: 10 minutes | Calories per portion: 49

Serves 4

1 cauliflower, cut into small florets

4 tbsp red wine vinegar

3 tbsp olive oil

1 garlic clove, finely chopped

a pinch of cayenne pepper

8 juniper berries, crushed

sea salt

Bring a pan of salted water to the boil, add the cauliflower and 3 tablespoons of the vinegar. Boil for 1 minute, then drain. Meanwhile, make a marinade with the rest of the ingredients (including the remaining vinegar). Mix in the cauliflower and serve.

NUTRITION PROFILE (per portion)
33% protein, 19% fat, 36% carbohydrate, 12% fibre

VITAMINS AND MINERALS (percentage of RDA)
Vitamin A 6%, C 57%, B1 17%, B5 10, B6 22, folate 35%, potassium 21%, calcium 6%, magnesium 8%, iron 7%, zinc 7%, manganese 17%

HEALTH BENEFITS
Helps maintain energy levels | regulates blood fat levels | antibiotic | benefits skin, muscles and joints

Golden Berry and Pumpkin Fritters

Preparation and cooking time: 30 minutes | Calories per portion: 211

Serves 4

500g/1lb 2oz pumpkin, peeled, deseeded
and cubed

50g/1¾oz golden berries

125g/4½oz/1 cup plain/all-purpose flour,
plus extra if needed

2 tsp baking powder

½ tsp sea salt

1 egg, beaten

milk, if needed

corn oil, for shallow-frying

Steam the pumpkin pieces for about 5 minutes, or until soft. Leave to stand in a colander for a few minutes. Mix all the other ingredients well (adding a little milk if the mixture seems too dry, or a little extra flour if it seems too wet), then stir in the pumpkin pieces.

Cover the bottom of a frying pan with about 1cm/½in oil and place over a medium-high heat. Once the oil is hot and sizzling, drop a tablespoonful of batter into the pan. Fry until golden on both sides and the fritter has a spongy consistency. Drain on paper towels and keep warm while you cook the remaining batter. Serve hot.

Tip: These fritters also make a delicious dessert served with a little cinnamon sugar or caramel sauce.

NUTRITION PROFILE (per portion)
14% protein, 42% fat, 40% carbohydrate, 4% fibre

VITAMINS AND MINERALS (percentage of RDA)
Vitamin A 14%, D 4%, E 26%, C 25%, B1 34%, B2 7%, B3 16%, B5 16%, B6 14%, B12 13%, folate 18%, biotin 10%, potassium 14%, calcium 11%, magnesium 14%, iron 15%, zinc 14%, copper 17%, manganese 54%, selenium 6%, iodine 4%

HEALTH BENEFITS
Promotes healthy skin | may dampen allergic reactions and inhibit the growth of cancer cells

Red Cabbage and Cranberries

Danes love tradition, and no Danish Christmas is complete without sweetened red cabbage! It first appeared in a recipe book written in 1888 (under the rather grand title 'chou rouge á la danoise'), and I still remember the sweet and sour smell of this lovely dish filling the house on Christmas Eve as my mother prepared our very traditional Christmas dinner. The berries were added to brighten up the colour, and gave a distinctive sweet sharpness to the taste. As in every other self-respecting Danish home, Christmas dinner was served at 6 o'clock sharp, and always consisted of a roast, boiled potatoes, sugared potatoes, apples, prunes and, of course, sweetened red cabbage. With every cooker in the land toiling under the same burden, power cuts were frequent between 5–6pm on Christmas Eve…

Preparation and cooking time: 1 hour 30 minutes | Calories per portion: 115

Serves 6

500g/1lb 2oz red cabbage, finely chopped

100ml/3½fl oz/scant ½ cup red wine vinegar

1 tsp sea salt

1 cooking/baking apple, peeled, cored and diced

100g/3½oz fresh or dried cranberries or lingonberries, rinsed

100ml/3½fl oz/scant ½ cup cranberry juice

100g/3½oz/½ cup raw cane sugar, plus extra if needed

Heat the cabbage in a heavy saucepan with the vinegar and salt. Bring to the boil, then turn down the heat and simmer, covered, for 1 hour. Add the apple, cranberries, cranberry juice and sugar. Heat through and simmer very gently for 10–15 minutes. Add a little more sugar if necessary for a delicate sweet and sour taste. Serve hot or cold.

NUTRITION PROFILE (per portion)
4% protein, 2% fat, 87% carbohydrate, 6% fibre

VITAMINS AND MINERALS (percentage of RDA)
Vitamin C 81%, B6 8%, folate 19%, potassium 15%, calcium 8%, iron 5%

HEALTH BENEFITS
Combined liver detox and natural antibiotic | may help strengthen cell walls and improve
the health of mucous membranes

MAIN COURSES

Savoury Spinach Parcels

Preparation and cooking time: 30 minutes | Calories per portion: 412

Serves 4

1 tbsp olive oil, plus extra for greasing

300g/10½oz chicken breast fillet, or tofu, sliced

500g/1lb 2oz fresh spinach, rinsed

200g/7oz pitted dried jujube berries

100g/3½oz cream cheese

100g/3½oz mozzarella cheese, torn

250g/9oz ready-rolled puff pastry

sea salt and freshly ground black pepper

Preheat the oven to 200°C/400°F/Gas 6 and grease a baking sheet. Heat the oil in a large, heavy saucepan. Add the chicken slices and fry, stirring, for a few minutes until cooked through. Add the spinach and the jujube berries with a pinch of salt and stir gently until the spinach starts to wilt. Remove from the heat and leave to cool a little, then add the cheeses and season with salt and pepper.

Meanwhile, cut the ready-rolled pastry into four 12cm/4½in squares and place on the prepared baking sheet. Put a spoonful of filling in the middle of each square. Dab the edges of the squares with cold water. Bring the corners of the pastry to the centre and press together along the edges to make 4 ridges radiating from the centre, sealing the parcel. Bake for 15 minutes, or until golden brown.

Best served with mashed potato, steamed carrots and peas and a gravy or, for a lighter meal, serve with a green salad.

NUTRITION PROFILE (per portion)
25% protein, 54% fat, 19% carbohydrate, 2% fibre

VITAMINS AND MINERALS (percentage of RDA)
Vitamin A 168%, D 5%, E 16%, C 54%, B1 20%, B2 19%, B3 63%, B5 20%, B6 40%, folate 58%, biotin 4%, potassium 42%, calcium 33%, magnesium 21%, iron 19%, copper 14%, manganese 33%, selenium 20%, iodine 6%

HEALTH BENEFITS
High in antioxidants and vitamin A | benefits eyes and skin | helps relieve stress | increases stamina | protects against infection

Moroccan Tajine

Preparation and cooking time: about 2 hours | Calories per portion: 412

Serves 4

1 tbsp olive oil

1 red onion, sliced

400g/14oz lamb fillet or seitan, cubed

250g/9oz/1¾ cups cooked chickpeas

1 tsp ground cumin

1 tsp ground coriander

1 tsp grated root ginger

2 cinnamon sticks, broken

1 tsp turmeric

1 carrot, sliced

3 red chillies, deseeded and sliced

2 sweet potatoes, peeled and cut into chunks

400g/14oz butternut squash, peeled and
cut into chunks

20 pitted dried jujube berries, rinsed

50g/1¾oz/heaped ½ cup flaked/sliced
almonds

sea salt and freshly ground black pepper

Heat the oil gently in a tajine or large saucepan, add the onion and fry until just soft. Add the lamb and fry until browned. Stir in the chickpeas and spices and heat through. Add the vegetables and jujubes in layers. Pour in just enough water to cover the vegetables and season with salt and pepper. Cover, bring to the boil, then reduce the heat to low and simmer gently until the vegetables are soft and the lamb is tender, about 1 hour 30 minutes. Meanwhile, toast the almonds in a frying pan until just golden, then sprinkle over the tajine to serve.

Couscous is the perfect partner for this lightly spiced tajine.

NUTRITION PROFILE (per portion)
23% protein, 44% fat, 28% carbohydrate, 5% fibre

VITAMINS AND MINERALS (percentage of RDA)
Vitamin A 124%, D 6%, E 37%, C 85%, B1 34%, B2 19%, B3 33%, B5 23%, B6 36%, folate 62%, biotin 4%, potassium 53%, calcium 18%, magnesium 38%, iron 38%, zinc 47%, copper 51%, manganese 58%, selenium 8%, iodine 4%

HEALTH BENEFITS
Rich, nourishing and healing | helps combat stress and aids convalescence

Rose Hip-Marinated Chicken with Blueberry Salad

Preparation and cooking time: 30 minutes, plus 30 minutes marinating | Calories per portion: 269

Serves 4

300g/10½oz chicken breast fillet
   or firm tofu, sliced

1 tbsp olive oil

For the marinade

4 tbsp red wine vinegar

2 tbsp French mustard

4 garlic cloves

3 tbsp olive oil

2 tbsp orange juice

100g/3½oz rose hips, choke and seeds
   removed (*see* page 153)

1 tsp curry powder

sea salt and freshly ground black pepper

For the salad

4 large handfuls of salad leaves, shredded

200g/7oz/1⅓ cups green peas, blanched

200g/7oz blueberries

50g/1¾oz/heaped ⅓ cup pecan nuts

Blend all the marinade ingredients to a paste. Reserve half the marinade to use later as a dressing for the salad.

Put the sliced chicken in a non-metallic bowl and pour over the remaining marinade. Cover and leave to marinate in the refrigerator for at least 30 minutes.

Preheat the oven to 160°C/315°F/Gas 2–3. Fry the chicken slices in the oil for a few minutes until brown on both sides, then transfer to a baking dish and bake for 10 minutes, or until cooked through.

Meanwhile, combine the salad ingredients in a large bowl. Top with the cooked chicken and drizzle with the reserved marinade dressing.

Serve with ciabatta bread.

Tip: Jujube berries or persimmons can be substituted for the rose hips.

NUTRITION PROFILE (per portion)
35% protein, 41% fat, 19% carbohydrate, 5% fibre

VITAMINS AND MINERALS (percentage of RDA)
Vitamin A 13%, E 15%, C 113%, B1 38%, B2 10%, B3 68%, B5 24%, B6 37%, folate 19%, potassium 31%, calcium 7%, magnesium 17%, iron 17%, zinc 15%, copper 18%, manganese 43%, selenium 20%

HEALTH BENEFITS
Nourishing | high in antioxidants | helps stimulate the immune system | aids wound healing and iron absorption | promotes steady energy release

Chinese Stir-Fry with Jujube and Goji Berries

Preparation and cooking time: 30 minutes, plus 20 minutes marinating | Calories per portion: 281

Serves 4

300g/10½oz chicken breast fillet or firm tofu, cut into chunks

2 tbsp sesame oil

2 spring onions/scallions, sliced diagonally

125g/4½oz mange tout/snow peas, kept whole

125g/4½oz baby corn, halved lengthways

250g/9oz Chinese cabbage, finely sliced

200g/7oz red or yellow pepper, finely sliced

50g/1¾oz pitted dried jujube berries, chopped

2 tbsp dried goji berries

1 bunch of coriander/cilantro leaves or mint, chopped

For the marinade

1 tbsp olive oil

juice and zest of 2 limes

2cm/¾in piece of red chilli, thinly sliced

2cm/¾in piece of root ginger, finely grated

2cm/¾in piece of lemongrass, finely sliced from the base

1 tbsp coriander seeds, crushed

1 tsp clear honey or syrup

1 tbsp sesame seeds

2 tbsp tamari soy sauce

sea salt and freshly ground black pepper

Combine all the ingredients for the marinade in a non-metallic dish. Add the chicken (or tofu), mix well, cover and leave to marinate in the refrigerator for at least 20 minutes while you prepare the rest of the ingredients.

Heat the sesame oil in a wok or large frying pan, add the marinated chicken and fry until crisp and golden, put to one side of the pan, then add the rest of the ingredients, one at a time, with a little more oil if needed and making sure to keep the temperature quite high. Stir-fry for a couple of minutes. Add the rest of the marinade mixture, bring to a boil and heat through. Sprinkle with the coriander/cilantro to serve.

This is best served in the traditional manner with rice or noodles.

Tip: You can replace the jujube berries with rose hips or chopped persimmon.

NUTRITION PROFILE (per portion)
36% protein, 41% fat, 20% carbohydrate, 5% fibre

VITAMINS AND MINERALS (percentage of RDA)
Vitamin A 44%, C 147%, B1 25%, B2 16%, B3 66%, B5 19%, B6 56%, folate 34%, biotin 3%, potassium 36%, calcium 17%, magnesium 19%, iron 28%, copper 21%, zinc 13%, selenium 26%

HEALTH BENEFITS
An energizing 'qi tonic' that helps stimulate circulation and improves immune response | benefits eyes, blood and skin

Mountain Berry Game Supreme

This is a modern version of a traditional Pyrenean dish. Tempeh makes a satisfying and nourishing vegetarian alternative to game.

Preparation and cooking time: 1 hour | Calories per portion: 199

Serves 4

2 grouse or partridges (about 500g/1lb 2oz total weight), or 500g/1lb 2oz tempeh

1 tbsp olive oil

250g/9oz mushrooms, preferably cèpes, sliced

2 carrots, roughly chopped

2 shallots, roughly chopped

10 juniper berries

1 small bunch of thyme, or 2 tsp dried thyme

1 small bunch of marjoram, or 2 tsp dried marjoram

300ml/10½fl oz/1¼ cups vegetable stock

200ml/7fl oz/scant 1 cup single/light almond cream

100g/3½oz redcurrants, rinsed and stalks removed

100g/3½oz elderberries, rinsed and stalks removed

sea salt and freshly ground black pepper

raw cane sugar, to taste

Divide each bird in two by cutting through the chest lengthways to make 4 pieces, each consisting of chest and a leg. Cut the legs and chests in two again, so you end up with 8 pieces. (If you are using tempeh, cut into 16 chunks.) Dry the pieces with paper towels and season.

Heat the oil in a large pan or casserole dish, then add the meat together with the mushrooms, carrots, shallots, juniper berries, thyme and marjoram. Fry over a gentle heat until the meat is golden. Pour in the vegetable stock, turn up the heat and bring to the boil, then turn down the heat, cover and simmer gently for 30–40 minutes, or until the meat is tender. Stir in the cream and the berries. Heat through again, taking care not to let the liquid boil, and adjust the seasoning.

Serve with a green salad, rice and Cloudberry Chutney (see page 180).

NUTRITION PROFILE (per portion)
42% protein, 39% fat, 14% carbohydrate, 5% fibre

VITAMINS AND MINERALS (percentage of RDA)
Vitamin A 56%, D 19%, E 7%, C 22%, B1 21%, B2 56%, B3 43%, B5 14%, B6 41%, folate 21%, biotin 2%, potassium 31%, calcium 14%, magnesium 11%, iron 37%, zinc 16%, selenium 32%

HEALTH BENEFITS
Low calorie | may ease rheumatic complaints and sore joints | good for digestion | helps combat infection | supports the immune system

Breast of Duck with Roast Potatoes and Redcurrant Sauce

Duck is a rich meat best served with a sharp sauce, such as redcurrant, which has excellent digestive properties. Nut cutlets are a good vegetarian alternative, cooked alongside the potatoes in the oven.

Preparation and cooking time: 1 hour | Calories per portion: 403

Serves 4

2 duck breasts (about 340g/12oz total weight), skin on, or 4 nut cutlets

4 garlic cloves, finely chopped

2 tbsp olive oil

500g/1lb 2oz potatoes, scrubbed and cut into small wedges

sea salt and freshly ground black pepper

For the redcurrant sauce

1 tbsp olive oil

2 shallots, finely chopped

3 garlic cloves, crushed

250ml/9fl oz/1 cup red wine

finely grated zest and juice of 1 orange

1 rosemary sprig

1 tsp tomato purée/paste

250g/9oz redcurrants, rinsed and stalks removed

1 tbsp raw cane sugar

Preheat the oven to 220°C/425°F/Gas 7. Using a sharp knife, score the duck skin, taking care not to cut into the meat. Rub the garlic into the scored skin, then sprinkle both sides of the duck breast with salt and pepper. Fry in a dry frying pan over a high heat for 2–5 minutes, skin-side down, until the fat melts and the skin becomes crunchy. Turn over and fry on the other side for about 30 seconds, then transfer to a roasting tray and leave to one side.

Heat the oil in another roasting tray in the oven until hot, then add the potato wedges, making sure they are well coated. Season with salt and pepper. Place the duck and the potatoes on the top shelf of the oven. After 7 minutes (for rare meat), or 10 minutes (for more well done), remove the duck from the oven and leave it to rest, covered, for at least 10 minutes. Leave the potatoes to cook through for another 10–15 minutes, or until golden brown, while you make the sauce.

To make the sauce, heat the oil in a frying pan and gently sauté the shallots and garlic. Add the wine, orange zest and juice, rosemary and tomato purée/paste, then cook until the liquid has reduced by half. Add the redcurrants and the sugar and heat through, stirring, until the redcurrants have burst and released their juices into the sauce.

Slice the duck breasts in half at an angle before serving half a breast per person with the potato wedges and redcurrant sauce.

NUTRITION PROFILE (per portion)
32% protein, 34% fat, 28% carbohydrate, 5% fibre

VITAMINS AND MINERALS (percentage of RDA)
Vitamin E 12%, C 69%, B1 73%, B2 34%, B3 33%, B5 25%, B6 33%, B12 38%, folate 39%, biotin 6%, potassium 52%, calcium 7%, magnesium 17%, iron 55%, zinc 16%, copper 62%, manganese 18%, selenium 34%

HEALTH BENEFITS
Rich and nourishing | benefits skin, energy levels and memory

Greek Cutlets with Blackberry Sauce

Preparation and cooking time: 1 hour, plus 1 hour marinating | Calories per portion: 403

Serves 4

8 lamb or tofu cutlets

For the marinade

200ml/7fl oz/scant 1 cup tomato ketchup

juice of 1 or 2 lemons (about 3 tbsp)

6 garlic cloves

1 tbsp mustard

1 tbsp olive oil

3 tbsp thyme leaves

1 tbsp paprika

½ tsp cayenne pepper

For the tzatziki

250ml/9fl oz/1 cup plain soy yogurt

1 cucumber, peeled, grated and drained

2 garlic cloves, crushed

1 tbsp olive oil

1 tbsp chopped mint leaves

For the potatoes

1kg/2lb 4oz potatoes, scrubbed and cut into wedges

2 tbsp olive oil

juice of 2 lemons

1 tsp dried thyme

1 tsp paprika

sea salt

For the blackberry sauce

500g/1lb 2oz blackberries

2 tbsp raw cane sugar

50g/1¾oz vegetable margarine

1 tbsp plain/all-purpose flour

Mix together all the ingredients for the marinade in a non-metallic dish. Add the cutlets, cover and leave to marinate in the refrigerator for at least 1 hour. In a separate bowl, mix together all the ingredients for the tzatziki, cover and refrigerate until needed.

Preheat the oven to 200°C/400°F/Gas 6. Rinse and dry the potato wedges. Place them in a roasting pan, drizzle with the oil, add the lemon juice, thyme and paprika, sprinkle with salt and roast for about 30 minutes until crisp and golden.

Meanwhile, rinse the blackberries, place in a bowl and and shake over the sugar. Melt the margarine in a saucepan and let it sizzle for a minute, then stir in the flour to make a smooth paste. Keep stirring while adding 500ml/17fl oz/2 cups water to make a thickish sauce. Gently fold in the blackberries and heat through, adding a little salt to taste, but avoid stirring too much or the berries will break up. Keep the sauce warm while you cook the cutlets.

Put the lamb cutlets on a grill/broiler rack, drizzle with the remaining marinade and grill/broil for about 5 minutes on each side until cooked through and golden. Serve immediately with the potatoes, tzatziki and blackberry sauce.

NUTRITION PROFILE (per portion)
20% protein, 39% fat, 37% carbohydrate, 4% fibre

VITAMINS AND MINERALS (percentage of RDA)
Vitamin A 27%, D 6%, E 27%, C 43%, B1 65%, B2 18%, B3 38%, B5 26%, B6 66%, folate 45%, biotin 4%, potassium 54%, calcium 15%, magnesium 20%, iron 45%, zinc 29%, copper 31%, selenium 7%, iodine 6%

HEALTH BENEFITS
Encourages steady energy release and concentration | immune booster | antioxidant and anti-inflammatory | benefits blood and circulation

Berry Moussaka

The berries provide a fresh contrast to the other ingredients, lifting the flavour of this traditional favourite. I recommend serving it with new potatoes, fresh bread and a green salad.

Preparation and cooking time: 1 hour | Calories per portion: 317

Serves 4

100g/3½oz redcurrants, rinsed and stalks removed

50g/1¾oz fresh cranberries, rinsed

1 tsp raw cane sugar, plus extra to taste

1 large aubergine/eggplant, thinly sliced

3–4 tbsp olive oil

1 tsp sea salt

250g/9oz minced/ground lamb, or finely chopped seitan

2 red onions, finely chopped

2 garlic cloves, crushed

1 red pepper, deseeded and finely chopped

250g/9oz mushrooms, sliced

1 bay leaf

2 thyme sprigs, or 2 tsp dried thyme

100g/3½oz tomato purée/paste

freshly ground black pepper

For the topping

2–3 eggs or 100g/3½oz silken tofu

100ml/3½fl oz/scant ½ cup plain soy yogurt

Put the berries in a bowl, sprinkle the sugar over and leave to one side.

Preheat the oven to 200°C/400°F/Gas 6. Toss the aubergine/eggplant slices in 1 tablespoon of the oil, the salt and a little black pepper. Heat a little of the remaining oil in a heavy frying pan, add the aubergine/eggplant slices and fry on both sides over a medium heat until golden. Remove and leave to one side, then heat a little more oil in the pan and fry the lamb for about 10 minutes until browned, then leave to one side.

Heat 1 tablespoon of the oil in a large casserole dish. Soften the onions, garlic and red pepper for 2–3 minutes. Add the mushrooms and stir-fry over a medium-high heat until they release their moisture. Add the bay leaf, thyme and tomato purée/paste. Heat through, then add the browned meat and the berries. Season to taste with sugar, salt and pepper. Cover and leave to simmer gently over a low heat while you prepare the topping by beating together the eggs (or tofu), yogurt, salt and pepper in a bowl.

Line an ovenproof dish with half of the aubergine/eggplant slices, add the filling, then lay the remaining aubergine/eggplant slices over the top and finish off by pouring over the topping. Make a few holes here and there to allow the topping to seep down into the filling. Bake for about 30 minutes, or until the topping has set and is golden. Serve hot.

NUTRITION PROFILE (per portion)
28% protein, 50% fat, 18% carbohydrate, 4% fibre

VITAMINS AND MINERALS (percentage of RDA)
Vitamin A 40%, D 13%, E 20%, C 86%, B1 19%, B2 33%, B3 39%, B5 36%, B6 40%, folate 33%, biotin 28%, potassium 45%, calcium 11%, magnesium 13%, iron 37%, zinc 36%, selenium 20%, iodine 12%

HEALTH BENEFITS
Antioxidant | increases immunity and helps repair damaged tissues | combats urinary tract infections | promotes stable energy levels

Shepherd's Pie

Preparation and cooking time: 1 hour | Calories per portion: 364

Serves 4

500g/1lb 2oz minced/ground lamb, or
   250g/9oz cooked lentils

1–2 tbsp olive oil, plus extra for greasing

1 large onion, finely chopped

3 garlic cloves, crushed

2 carrots, grated

2 celery stalks, finely sliced

1 tsp curry powder

2 bay leaves

2 thyme sprigs, or 2 tsp dried thyme

400g/14oz tomatoes, chopped

200ml/7fl oz/scant 1 cup vegetable stock

1 tbsp tomato purée/paste

100g/3½oz aronia berries

sea salt and freshly ground black pepper

For the mashed potato topping

1kg/2lb 4oz potatoes, quartered

55ml/1¾fl oz/scant ¼ cup soy milk

100g/3½oz vegetable margarine

sea salt and freshly ground black pepper

paprika, for sprinkling

Brown the lamb in a little oil in a frying pan over a high heat, then leave to one side. Heat the oil in a separate large pan, add the onion and sauté until it starts to soften, then add the garlic, carrots, celery, curry powder and herbs. Sauté for another 5 minutes or so until the vegetables just start to brown. Stir in the tomatoes, vegetable stock, tomato purée/paste, cooked lamb and the aronia berries. Bring gently to the boil and simmer for another 5 minutes. Season to taste.

Meanwhile, put the potatoes in a pan of salted water. Bring to the boil, then turn the heat down and simmer for about 15 minutes until tender. Drain them well, then mash with the milk and margarine. Season to taste.

Preheat the oven to 210°C/415°F/Gas 6–7 and grease a 2l/70fl oz/8½ cups ovenproof dish. Spoon the filling into the dish, then cover it with the mashed potato and a sprinkling of paprika. Bake in the middle of the oven for 15 minutes, or until the mashed potato is golden.

Tips: You can substitute the aronia berries with jujubes or almost any other berry. If you use very acidic berries, you may need to adjust the flavour of the dish by adding a little sugar. You can use any kind of lentils, but beluga lentils are particularly good for shepherd's pie.

NUTRITION PROFILE (per portion)
11% protein, 37% fat, 47% carbohydrate, 5% fibre

VITAMINS AND MINERALS (percentage of RDA)
Vitamin A 78%, E 22%, C 51%, B1 51%, B2 9%, B3 15%, B5 16%, B6 79%, folate 52%, biotin 4%, potassium 59%, calcium 10%, magnesium 17%, iron 36%, zinc 15%, copper 33%, manganese 37%, selenium 32%, iodine 5%

HEALTH BENEFITS
Strongly antioxidant | helps maintain good energy levels | helps combat stress

Venison Bourguignon

Preparation and cooking time: 1 hour | Calories per portion: 368

Serves 4

2 tbsp olive oil

250g/9oz roebuck venison fillet, or
   250g/9oz tempeh, cut into chunks

200g/7oz small onions, peeled and left whole

4 garlic cloves, roughly chopped

350g/12oz fresh or tinned sweet chestnuts,
   or 150g/5½oz dried chestnuts, soaked

250g/9oz button mushrooms, kept whole

3 tbsp plain/all-purpose flour

2 bay leaves

1 tsp dried thyme

1 tbsp finely chopped parsley

250ml/9fl oz/1 cup vegetable stock

2 tbsp tomato purée/paste

250ml/9fl oz/1 cup red wine

250g/9oz damsons, halved and pitted

1 tsp honey, or to taste

sea salt and freshly ground black pepper

Preheat the oven to 180°C/350°F/Gas 4. Heat 1 tablespoon of the oil in a medium heavy pan and sear the roebuck fillet on each side for a minute or two until golden brown. Remove from the pan and leave to one side.

Heat the remaining oil in the same pan and gently sauté the onions, garlic, chestnuts and mushrooms until golden. Sprinkle with the flour, add the herbs and heat through, stirring continuously until everything is coated in flour and herbs. Remove the pan from the heat and add the stock together with the rest of the ingredients, including the browned venison. Season to taste, then transfer to a casserole dish, cover and cook in the middle of the oven for 40 minutes, or until tender, adding more stock if necessary. Serve hot, perhaps with rice and a green salad.

NUTRITION PROFILE (per portion)
25% protein, 19% fat, 48% carbohydrate, 6% fibre

VITAMINS AND MINERALS (percentage of RDA)
Vitamin A 7%, E 18%, C 15%, B1 41%, B2 34%, B3 53%, B5 34%, B6 65%, folate 23%, biotin 17%, potassium 57%, calcium 14%, magnesium 19%, iron 42%, zinc 30%, copper 79%, manganese 45%, selenium 23%, iodine 2%

HEALTH BENEFITS
Helps maintain good cholesterol levels | combats age-related tissue degeneration

Pasta with Walnut and Blackcurrant Pesto

Preparation and cooking time: 20 minutes | Calories per portion: 377

Serves 4

400g/14oz dried pasta

5 tbsp chopped walnuts

1 tsp sea salt

1 bunch of basil

1 tbsp olive oil, plus extra for cooking

2 garlic cloves

100g/3½oz blackcurrants, rinsed and stalks removed

Cook the pasta in a large saucepan of boiling salted water with a drop of oil for 10 minutes, or until al dente, then drain.

Meanwhile, blend all the other ingredients, except the blackcurrants, to make a coarse paste. Transfer the mixture to a small bowl, add the blackcurrants and stir well, crushing some of the berries into the sauce and leaving some whole. Put the drained pasta into a heated serving dish, mix in the blackcurrant pesto and serve immediately.

Serve with a green salad and some sliced tomatoes.

NUTRITION PROFILE (per portion)
15% protein, 28% fat, 53% carbohydrate, 4% fibre

VITAMINS AND MINERALS (percentage of RDA)
Vitamin A 9%, E 6%, C 53%, B1 76%, B2 10%, B3 32%, B5 14%, B6 29%, folate 16%, biotin 6%, potassium 24%, calcium 9%, magnesium 31%, iron 30%, zinc 28%, copper 56%, manganese 123%, selenium 24%, iodine 1%

HEALTH BENEFITS
Provides quick energy release | helps combat infections and reduce inflammation | protects heart and circulation

Spicy Falafel Burgers with Açai-Tahini Sauce

I prefer to use dried chickpeas, but you can save soaking and cooking time by using tinned or pre-cooked chickpeas.

Preparation and cooking time (dried chickpeas): 1 hour 20 minutes, plus soaking |
Calories per portion: 366

Serves 4

150g/5½oz/scant 1 cup dried chickpeas,
   soaked for at least 8 hours,
   or 300g/10½oz/1½ cups tinned
   chickpeas, drained and rinsed
1 small onion, quartered
2 garlic cloves
¼ red pepper, chopped
1 small red chilli pepper, chopped
1 small handful of parsley leaves
1 tsp paprika

½ tsp ground cardamom
½ tsp ground nutmeg
½ tsp ground cinnamon
1 tsp ground cumin
1 tsp ground coriander
½ tsp black pepper
1 tsp sea salt
1 tsp baking powder
olive oil, for shallow-frying

For the açai-tahini sauce

2 tbsp tahini (sesame seed paste)
2 garlic cloves, crushed
1 tbsp lemon juice

1 tsp powdered açai berries
½ tsp sea salt

To serve

4 sesame buns, sliced in half
4 lettuce leaves

2 tomatoes, thinly sliced
1 small onion, thinly sliced

Drain and rinse the chickpeas and put into a saucepan. Cover with cold water, bring to the boil over a high heat and boil for 10 minutes. Turn down the heat and leave to simmer for a further 45 minutes. Drain and leave to cool for 10 minutes.

Meanwhile, make the açai-tahini sauce by combining the tahini, garlic, lemon juice, açai powder and salt with enough water to make a smooth, creamy paste.

Combine all the remaining falafel ingredients (except the oil) with about 55ml/ 1¾fl oz/scant ¼ cup water in a blender or food processor and grind to a thick paste. Wet your hands and roll little handfuls of the mixture into 8 small balls. Flatten and shape into round patties and shallow-fry over a medium-high heat until golden.

Serve hot in burger buns with lettuce, tomato, onion and the açai-tahini sauce.

NUTRITION PROFILE (per portion)
17% protein, 30% fat, 47% carbohydrate, 6% fibre

VITAMINS AND MINERALS (percentage of RDA)
Vitamin A 33%, E 17%, C 58%, B1 41%, B2 14%, B3 18%, B5 17%, B6 33%, folate 61%, biotin 5%, potassium 38%, calcium 30%, magnesium 31%, iron 45%, zinc 23%, copper 60%, manganese 75%, selenium 10%

HEALTH BENEFITS
Nourishing | good source of unsaturated fat | an energy booster and blood sugar stabilizer | strengthens muscles, bones, skin, nails and hair

Golden Berry Nut Roast

Preparation and cooking time: 1 hour | Calories per portion: 377

Serves 4

4 tbsp olive oil

1 onion, chopped

250g/9oz mushrooms, sliced

5 spring onions/scallions, thinly sliced

1 celery stalk, finely sliced

1 tbsp plain/all-purpose flour, plus extra for
 dusting

300ml/10½fl oz/1¼ cups vegetable stock

120g/4¼oz/1 cup finely chopped
 hazelnuts, Brazil nuts and cashew nuts

1 apple, peeled, cored and diced

150g/5½oz/1¾ cups fresh breadcrumbs

1 tbsp soy sauce

2 tbsp finely chopped parsley and sage

1cm/½in piece of root ginger, peeled
 and grated

250g/9oz dried golden berries

sea salt and freshly ground black pepper

Preheat the oven to 200°C/400°F/Gas 6. Heat 1 tablespoon of the oil in a large, heavy saucepan and gently fry the onion until soft. Turn up the heat a little and add the mushrooms. Stir-fry until they release their moisture and turn slightly golden. Add the spring onions/scallions and celery and sauté for another minute, then sprinkle in the flour. Stir well until all the vegetables are coated. Pour in the stock, stirring all the time. Bring to the boil and simmer for a couple of minutes. Stir in the nuts, apple, breadcrumbs, soy sauce, herbs, ginger and golden berries. Mix well and season with salt and pepper.

Leave the mixture to cool a little, then pour it onto a floured board. Dust your hands with a little flour and shape the mixture to form a 'loaf' that will fit into a medium roasting pan. Pour the remaining oil into the roasting pan and heat in the oven. Place the nut loaf in the pan and bake for 35 minutes, basting with the oil from time to time.

Serve with potatoes, green vegetables and Gooseberry Sauce (see page 189).

NUTRITION PROFILE (per portion)
15% protein, 49% fat, 34% carbohydrate, 3% fibre

VITAMINS AND MINERALS (percentage of RDA)
Vitamin A 4%, E 26%, C 23%, B1 36%, B2 18%, B3 29%, B5 25%, B6 24%, folate 33%, biotin 30%, potassium 28%, calcium 13%, magnesium 26%, iron 26%, zinc 17%, manganese 60%, selenium 313%, iodine 3%

HEALTH BENEFITS
Rich in antioxidants and omega oils | helps lower blood cholesterol | reduces stress and restlessness | immunity booster | helps red blood cells to function properly

Rose Hip Risotto

Short-grain rice, such as Arborio, is the best to use here as a risotto should have a rich consistency, yet with the rice grains still separate and al dente. The addition of rose hips and pumpkin give this risotto a sunny appearance and a creamy taste with a sharp edge.

Preparation and cooking time: 45 minutes | Calories per portion: 307

Serves 4

1 tbsp olive oil

1 leek, finely chopped

3 garlic cloves, crushed

1 Hokkaido pumpkin or butternut squash, peeled, deseeded and cubed

300g/10½oz/1½ cups risotto rice

800ml/28fl oz/scant 3½ cups hot vegetable stock

100g/3½oz rose hips, rinsed, trimmed and deseeded (see page 153)

1 tbsp dried oregano

sea salt and freshly ground black pepper

1 tbsp Parmesan cheese, grated, or brewer's yeast flakes, to serve

Heat the oil in a large, heavy saucepan. Add the leek, garlic and pumpkin and sauté over a gentle heat for 3–5 minutes. Stir in the rice and make sure it is heated through and coated in oil before you add a ladleful of stock. Simmer, stirring from time to time, until the liquid has been absorbed. Continue to add the hot stock a ladleful at a time until all the liquid has been absorbed and the rice is al dente, about 30 minutes. Add the rose hips and oregano, heat through and serve with freshly grated Parmesan.

NUTRITION PROFILE (per portion)
9% protein, 17% fat, 69% carbohydrate, 5% fibre

VITAMINS AND MINERALS (percentage of RDA)
Vitamin A 30%, E 32%, C 137%, B1 66%, B2 7%, B3 22%, B5 15%, B6 15%, folate 31%, biotin 2%, potassium 31%, calcium 16%, magnesium 27%, iron 22%, zinc 16%, copper 55%, manganese 88%, selenium 11%

HEALTH BENEFITS
High in vitamin C | boosts healing and energy levels | helps regulate cholesterol and blood sugar levels, | protects against heart disease and cancer

Goji Pilaf

A pilaf is a rice dish cooked in stock. The name is derived from the Sanskrit *pulaka*, meaning 'shrivelled grain', and the practice may have started as a way of adding flavour to old rice. Try replacing the goji berries with barberries, which are also a traditional ingredient in pilaf. Barberries look like goji berries but are smaller and give a slightly sharp, tart flavour.

Preparation and cooking time: 35 minutes | Calories per portion: 377

Serves 4

1 tbsp olive oil
250g/9oz/1⅓ cups long-grain rice
750ml/26fl oz/3 cups vegetable stock
100g/3½oz dried goji berries
200g/7oz dried mulberries
5 cardamom pods, lightly crushed
1 tsp turmeric
1 cinnamon stick
1 orange, unpeeled, cut into small thin segments
100g/3½oz/¾ cup almonds, chopped and toasted
sea salt and freshly ground black pepper

Heat the oil in a large sauté pan and stir-fry the rice for 1 minute. Add the stock, berries and spices. Bring to the boil, then turn the heat down to low, cover and simmer very gently for 25 minutes, or until all the liquid is absorbed. Season to taste, then stir in the orange segments. Heat through, sprinkle with almonds and serve hot or cold.

NUTRITION PROFILE (per portion)
13% protein, 36% fat, 47% carbohydrate, 4% fibre

VITAMINS AND MINERALS (percentage of RDA)
Vitamin E 44%, C 22%, B1 26%, B2 15%, B3 21%, B5 16%, B6 22%, folate 18%, biotin 26%, potassium 21%, calcium 14%, magnesium 35%, iron 37%, zinc 17%, copper 38%, selenium 21%

HEALTH BENEFITS
Benefits circulation and immune function | aids recovery after cancer treatment | may help prevent neurodegenerative problems and hormone-related cancers

DESSERTS AND BAKING

Scandinavian Fruit Dessert (Rødgrød Med Fløde)

Preparation and cooking time: 30 minutes, plus chilling | Calories per portion: 215

Serves 8

1kg/2lb 4oz mixed berries (strawberries, redcurrants, raspberries,
blackcurrants), rinsed and stalks removed
250g/9oz rhubarb, rinsed and chopped
250g/9oz/1¼ cups caster/granulated sugar, plus 1 tbsp for sprinkling
2.5cm/1in vanilla pod/bean
1–2 tbsp potato flour dissolved in a little cold water

Put the berries and rhubarb into a saucepan with 200ml/7fl oz/scant 1 cup water, the sugar and the vanilla pod/bean. Bring to the boil gently, cover with a lid and simmer over a low heat for 10–15 minutes, stirring from time to time. Remove from the heat and mix in the dissolved potato flour. Pour into a serving bowl and sprinkle with a thin layer of sugar to prevent a skin forming on the surface. Once cool, cover and chill in the refrigerator for about 30 minutes before serving.

Serve with cream or vanilla ice cream.

NUTRITION PROFILE (per portion)
5% protein, 1% fat, 87% carbohydrate, 7% fibre

VITAMINS AND MINERALS (percentage of RDA)
Vitamin C 161%, folate 11%, potassium 27%, calcium 12%, iron 13%

HEALTH BENEFITS
Antioxidant | high vitamin C content | may help reduce inflammation, blood pressure and blood cholesterol levels

Rose Hip Soup

Packed full of vitamins, rose hip soup is a traditional Swedish dessert, usually eaten cold with crème frâiche and little round vanilla cookies called *kammerjunkere*. In modern Scandinavian cuisine, it is also served hot and as a first course.

Preparation and cooking time: 40 minutes, plus chilling | Calories per portion: 177

Serves 4

750g/1lb 10oz rose hips, rinsed, trimmed and deseeded (see below)

100g/3½oz/½ cup raw cane sugar

1 tbsp lemon juice

1 tbsp potato flour dissolved in a little cold water

Place the rose hips in a saucepan with 1l/35fl oz/4¼ cups water and bring to the boil. Turn the heat down to low and simmer, covered, for about 15 minutes until the rose hips are tender. Remove from the heat and blend to a smooth purée. Stir in the sugar, return the pan to the heat and bring back to the boil. Turn off the heat, add the lemon juice and the dissolved potato flour a little at a time, stirring continuously, until you have a smooth consistency. Once cool, cover and chill in the refrigerator for about 30 minutes before serving.

Serve with sweet croûtons and crème frâiche or whipped cream.

Tip: The easiest way to remove rose hip seeds is to cut the berries in half and scoop them out using a teaspoon. Rinse well after.

NUTRITION PROFILE (per portion)
3% protein, 1% fat, 95% carbohydrate, 1% fibre

VITAMINS AND MINERALS (percentage of RDA)
Vitamin A 43%, E 39%, C 426%, B1 7%, B2 12%, B5 11%, potassium 19%, calcium 17%, magnesium 15%, iron 7%

HEALTH BENEFITS
Extremely rich in vitamin C | provides natural energy and an immunity boost | enhances wound healing | inhibits inflammation | slows cancer cell growth

Elderberry Soup

Preparation and cooking time: 35 minutes | Calories per portion: 127

Serves 4

1kg/2lb 4oz elderberries, rinsed and stalks removed

2 apples, peeled and cut into slices

1 cinnamon stick

peel of 1 unwaxed lemon

200g/7oz/1 cup raw cane sugar

2 tbsp potato flour, dissolved in a little cold water

Bring 1.5l/52fl oz/6 cups water to the boil and add the berries, apples, cinnamon and lemon peel. Turn the heat down to low and simmer for 20 minutes. Strain off the juice through a sieve/fine-mesh strainer into a container, then pour the juice back into the saucepan. Add the sugar and boil through, stirring, until it is dissolved. Turn off the heat and gradually stir in the dissolved potato flour a little at a time, stirring continuously, until you have a smooth consistency. Serve hot, or cool, cover and chill in the refrigerator for about 30 minutes to serve chilled.

Serve with cream, granola, croûtons, apple or pear slices.

NUTRITION PROFILE (per portion)
3% protein, 3% fat, 83% carbohydrate, 11% fibre

VITAMINS AND MINERALS (percentage of RDA)
Vitamin A 6%, C 33%, B1 6%, B2 5%, B3 6%, B6 15%, folate 8%, potassium 16%, calcium 6%, iron 13%

HEALTH BENEFITS
Low calorie | helpful in the management of immune deficiency states and infections | benefits the lungs

Summer Berry Crumble

Preparation and cooking time: 30 minutes | Calories per portion: 315

Serves 4

1kg/2lb 4oz mixed loganberries, raspberries, boysenberries, dewberries or blackberries, rinsed

3 tbsp raw cane sugar

100g/3½oz/¾ cup plain/all-purpose flour

100g/3½oz/1 cup rolled oats

100g/3½oz/¾ cup hazelnuts, chopped

100g/3½oz vegetable margarine, diced, plus extra for greasing

4 tbsp maple syrup

Preheat the oven to 200°C/400°F/Gas 6. Mix the berries with the sugar and 2 tablespoons of the flour, then pour into a 23cm/9in greased ovenproof dish.

For the topping, mix the rest of the flour with the oats, hazelnuts and margarine. Spoon the mixture over the berries in an even layer. Drizzle with maple syrup and bake for 20 minutes, or until golden.

Serve with cream or yogurt.

NUTRITION PROFILE (per portion)
7% protein, 55% fat, 33% carbohydrate, 5% fibre

VITAMINS AND MINERALS (percentage of RDA)
Vitamin A 15%, D 23%, E 29%, C 22%, B1 18%, B6 12%, folate 26%, biotin 18%, potassium 16%, calcium 7%, magnesium 17%, zinc 13%

HEALTH BENEFITS
Nourishing and soothing | benefits the skin, nails, hair and eyes | antioxidant | may help lower LDL and cholesterol levels in the blood

Dewberry One-Crust Pie

Preparation and cooking time: 50 minutes, plus chilling | Calories per portion: 289

Serves 8

For the pastry dough

250g/9oz/2 cups plain/all-purpose flour

½ tsp sea salt

60g/2¼oz/⅓ cup caster/granulated sugar

125g/4½oz cold vegetable margarine, diced, plus extra for greasing

beaten egg or a little milk, for glazing

For the filling

500g/1lb 2oz dewberries

2 tbsp cornflour/cornstarch

125g/4½oz/⅔ cup raw cane sugar

Mix the flour, salt and sugar in a bowl. Add the margarine by chopping it into the flour with a knife and spoon until it forms small lumps. Continue to rub the fat into the flour with your fingers until the mixture resembles fine breadcrumbs. Gradually add about 70ml/2¼fl oz/¼ cup cold water to make a soft dough. Roll into a ball, wrap in cling film/plastic wrap and leave to chill in the refrigerator.

Preheat the oven to 200°C/400°F/Gas 6 and grease a 23cm/9in round baking pan. Mix the berries with the cornflour/cornstarch and sugar. Roll out the pastry and line the pan, letting the excess hang over the sides. Spread the berry mix over the pastry, then fold the edges in over the filling (they won't quite meet in the middle). Glaze with the egg or milk and bake for 20–30 minutes, or until golden. Serve hot.

NUTRITION PROFILE (per portion)
7% protein, 37% fat, 52% carbohydrate, 4% fibre

VITAMINS AND MINERALS (percentage of RDA)
Vitamin A 14%, D 22%, E 6%, C 23%, B1 14%, B2 5%, B3 11%, B5 7%, B6 13%, B12 6%, folate 17%, biotin 8%, potassium 12%, calcium 5%, magnesium 13%, iron 15%, zinc 10%, copper 23%, manganese 64%, selenium 5%

HEALTH BENEFITS
Antioxidant | anti-inflammatory | soothing to the digestive system

Mulberry Pie

Preparation and cooking time: 50 minutes, plus chilling | Calories per portion: 317

Serves 8

For the pastry dough

250g/9oz/2 cups plain/all-purpose flour

½ tsp sea salt

2 tbsp sugar

125g/4½oz cold vegetable margarine, diced, plus extra for greasing

a little milk or beaten egg for glazing

For the filling

450g/1lb mulberries, or 200g/7oz dried mulberries

200g/7oz/1 cup raw cane sugar

2 tbsp plain/all-purpose flour

1 tbsp grapeseed oil

Mix the flour, salt and sugar in a bowl. Add the margarine by chopping it into the flour with a knife and spoon until it forms small lumps. Continue to rub the fat into the flour with your fingers until the mixture resembles fine breadcrumbs. Gradually add about 70ml/2¼fl oz/¼ cup cold water to make a soft dough. Roll into a ball, wrap in cling film/plastic wrap and leave to chill in the refrigerator.

Preheat the oven to 200°C/400°F/Gas 6 and grease a 23cm/9in round baking pan. Mix the berries with the sugar and flour. Roll out two-thirds of the dough to fit the base and sides of the baking pan. Roll out the remaining third to make a lid. Scoop the berries into the base, drizzle with the oil and cover with the dough lid. Cut a few slits in the top, glaze with milk or egg and bake for 20–30 minutes until golden. Serve hot.

NUTRITION PROFILE (per portion)
6% protein, 36% fat, 55% carbohydrate, 3% fibre

VITAMINS AND MINERALS (percentage of RDA)
Vitamin A 13%, D 20%, C 12%, B1 14%, B3 12%, B6 12%, folate 17%, potassium 12%, magnesium 12%, iron 16%, zinc 10%

HEALTH BENEFITS
Helps maintain the health of skin and bones | protects agains cellular degeneration

Baked Stuffed Apples

Preparation and cooking time: 30 minutes | Calories per portion: 227

Serves 4

4 cooking/baking apples, cored but not peeled

100g/3½oz sea-buckthorn berries, rinsed

4 tsp sugar

4 dates, pitted and chopped

1 banana, peeled and mashed

1 tsp ground cinnamon

4 tbsp chopped almonds

4 tbsp maple syrup

Preheat the oven to 180°C/350°F/Gas 4. Score a line horizontally around the middle of each apple. Place the berries in a bowl and sprinkle with the sugar. Gently mix in the dates, banana and cinnamon, then stuff the mixture into the apple centres. Transfer the stuffed apples to a shallow ovenproof dish, sprinkle each one with the nuts and a spoonful of maple syrup. Bake for 20 minutes, or until the apples are cooked through.

Serve with extra maple syrup, whipped cream or crème fraîche.

NUTRITION PROFILE (per portion)
7% protein, 29% fat, 59% carbohydrate, 5% fibre

VITAMINS AND MINERALS (percentage of RDA)
Vitamin E 28%, C 87%, B2 29%, B3 91%, B6 26%, folate 9%, B12 44%, biotin 16%, potassium 24%, calcium 11%, magnesium 13%, iron 52%, zinc 12%

HEALTH BENEFITS
Encourages the healing of skin problems | useful in the management of colds, flu and general inflammation | benefits the nervous system

Damson Dessert

This tasty dessert is a cross between a pie and a sponge cake with a subtle yet distinctive flavour. It is delicious served with cream.

Preparation and cooking time: 1 hour | Calories per portion: 313

Serves 8

500g/1lb 2oz damsons, pitted   250g/9oz/1¼ cups raw cane sugar

For the cake sponge

100g/3½oz vegetable margarine, softened,   1 egg, beaten
  plus extra for greasing   100g/3½oz/¾ cup plain/all-purpose flour
100g/3½oz/½ cup raw cane sugar   2 tsp baking powder

Place the damsons and sugar in a heavy saucepan. Add enough water to just cover the fruit. Bring to the boil, then reduce the heat and simmer gently, covered, until soft. This will take about 15 minutes.

Meanwhile, beat the margarine with the sugar to make a smooth consistency, then beat in the egg. Sift the flour and baking powder into the mixture and gently fold in.

Preheat the oven to 180°C/350°F/Gas 4. Grease a 23cm/9in round cake pan, then pour in the damson mixture, followed by the batter. Bake in the middle of the oven for 30 minutes, or until risen. Leave to cool for 10 minutes. Loosen around the edges and invert onto a serving plate.

NUTRITION PROFILE (per portion)
4% protein, 28% fat, 66% carbohydrate, 2% fibre

VITAMINS AND MINERALS (percentage of RDA)
Vitamin A 16%, D 20%, E 5%, C 4%, B1 10%, B5 6%, B6 7%, B12 6%, folate 5%, biotin 4%, potassium 11%, calcium 6%, magnesium 6%, iron 8%, zinc 5%

HEALTH BENEFITS
Powerfully antioxidant | helps protect against age-related tissue degeneration

Persimmon Pudding

This sumptuous pudding has the texture of a soft sponge cake and a spicy flavour with a hint of caramel.

Preparation and cooking time: 1 hour 15 minutes | Calories per portion: 289

Serves 4

300g/10½oz persimmons, peeled and
  deseeded
200ml/7fl oz/scant 1 cup soy milk
100g/3½oz/½ cup raw cane sugar
125g/4½oz/1 cup plain/all-purpose flour

2 tsp baking powder
½ tsp ground cinnamon
½ tsp vanilla extract
a pinch of salt
50g/1¾oz/⅓ cup walnuts, chopped

Preheat the oven to 180°C/350°F/Gas 4 and grease a 23cm/9in round cake pan. Blend the persimmon pulp and pour into a mixing bowl. Stir in the milk and sugar. Sift in the flour and baking powder and fold in gently. Fold in the remaining ingredients.

Pour the mixture into the prepared pan and bake for 1 hour, or until a skewer inserted into the middle comes out clean. Leave to cool in the pan before turning out onto a wire/cooling rack or serving plate.

Serve warm with ice cream, whipped cream, crème fraîche or yogurt.

NUTRITION PROFILE (per portion)
10% protein, 24% fat, 62% carbohydrate, 4% fibre

VITAMINS AND MINERALS (percentage of RDA)
Vitamin A 11%, E 7%, C 14%, B1 17%, B2 14%, B3 12%, B5 7%, B6 12%, folate 14%, potassium 16%, calcium 7%, magnesium 17%, iron 12%, zinc 12%, selenium 31%

HEALTH BENEFITS
Energizing and immune booster | benefits the nerves, heart, blood and microcirculation

Honeyberry Cheesecake

If you don't have any honeyberries, this recipe works equally well with raspberries, blueberries, strawberries or redcurrants.

Preparation and cooking time: 1 hour | Calories per portion: 355

Serves 10

10 digestive biscuits/graham crackers, crushed

50g/1¾oz vegetable margarine, plus extra for greasing

600g/1lb 5oz cream cheese

3 tbsp plain/all-purpose flour

200g/7oz/1 cup raw cane sugar

2 eggs, beaten

150ml/5fl oz/⅔ cup plain yogurt

5 drops of vanilla extract

500g/1lb 2oz honeyberries, rinsed

3 tbsp maple syrup

Preheat the oven to 180°C/350°F/Gas 4. Grease the sides and base of a 23cm/9in round cake pan. Blend the biscuits/crackers with the margarine and press into the prepared pan. Bake for 5 minutes and leave to one side.

Meanwhile, put the cream cheese, flour, sugar, eggs, yogurt and vanilla in a bowl and beat to a light fluffy consistency. Gently fold in one-third of the honeyberries and pour the cream cheese and berry mixture on top of the base. Bake for 45 minutes, then leave to cool completely on a wire/cooling rack before removing from the pan.

Bring the remainder of the berries, reserving a few for decoration, to the boil with the maple syrup, then simmer gently, until the berries give off their juice and disintegrate a little. Decorate the cake with the reserved whole berries and serve with the sauce.

NUTRITION PROFILE (per portion)
5% protein, 65% fat, 29% carbohydrate, 1% fibre

VITAMINS AND MINERALS (percentage of RDA)
Vitamin A 26%, D 10%, E 9%, B2 9%, B12 13%, calcium 12%, iron 6%, zinc 6%, selenium 5%

HEALTH BENEFITS
Good for bones | benefits heart, circulation and digestion

Chilled Rice Pudding with Hot Cherry Sauce

This is a traditional Danish Christmas dessert, but you can eat it all year round. In Denmark, the tradition is to leave one almond whole, and whoever gets it wins a prize – usually a pig made of marzipan!

Preparation and cooking time: 1 hour, plus chilling | Calories per portion: 417

Serves 4

For the rice pudding

125g/4½oz/⅔ cup pudding rice, rinsed

1l/35fl oz/4¼ cups soy milk

1 vanilla pod/bean, split

4 tbsp golden caster sugar

400ml/14fl oz/1⅔ cups soy whipping or double/heavy cream

100g/3½oz/¾ cup almonds, blanched and chopped

For the cherry sauce

500g/1lb 2oz cherries, pitted

250g/9oz/1¼ cups golden caster/granulated sugar

100ml/3½fl oz/scant ½ cup port or rum

1 tbsp cornflour/cornstarch

1 tbsp lemon juice, or to taste

Place the rice in a heavy saucepan. Add the milk and the vanilla pod/bean and slowly bring to the boil. Reduce the heat, cover with a lid and simmer very gently, stirring occasionally, for about 30 minutes. Stir in the sugar and leave to one side to cool. Remove the vanilla pod/bean.

Whip the cream and fold it gently into the cooled rice together with the almonds. Cover and keep cool in the refrigerator until ready to serve.

For the sauce, bring the cherries, sugar and port to the boil in a saucepan. Turn the heat down to low and simmer for 10–15 minutes. Dissolve the cornflour/cornstarch in 2 tablespoons of cold water and add to the sauce, stirring constantly. Heat through and add lemon juice to taste.

Serve the rice pudding topped with the warm cherry sauce.

Tip: To remove the almond skins, cover them with boiling water and leave for a few minutes until the skin loosens and can be rubbed off.

NUTRITION PROFILE (per portion)
11% protein, 26% fat, 62% carbohydrate, 1% fibre

VITAMINS AND MINERALS (percentage of RDA)
Vitamin E 31%, C 9%, B1 12%, B2 30%, B6 9%, folate 15%, biotin 15%, potassium 21%, calcium 8%, magnesium 16%, iron 11%, zinc 10%

HEALTH BENEFITS
Nourishing with a calming effect | helps protect cells from the effects of environmental toxins | may help reduce susceptibility to heart disease and cancer

Blackberry Raw Dessert

Preparation time: 10 minutes | Calories per portion: 199

Serves 4

2 avocados, peeled and pitted

3 bananas, peeled

1 mango, peeled, pitted and cut into small chunks

1 tbsp açai berry pulp

100g/3½oz blackberries, rinsed

Blend the avocados with the bananas to make a purée and place in a serving dish. Gently mix the mango chunks into the purée. Sprinkle with the açai berry pulp, top with the blackberries and serve.

NUTRITION PROFILE (per portion)
7% protein, 29% fat, 56% carbohydrate, 8% fibre

VITAMINS AND MINERALS (percentage of RDA)
Vitamin A 12%, E 19%, C 51%, B1 8%, B2 10%, B3 10%, B5 16%, B6 28%, folate 25%, potassium 31%, magnesium 13%, iron 8%

HEALTH BENEFITS
Energy-rich | high in vitamin C | immunity booster | protects blood vessel linings

Gooseberry Fool

Preparation and cooking time: 25 minutes, plus chilling | Calories per portion: 167

Serves 4

500g/1lb 2oz gooseberries, topped and tailed

4 tbsp raw cane sugar, plus extra to taste

300ml/10½fl oz/1¼ cups soy topping cream, double/heavy cream or Greek yogurt

Place the gooseberries in a heavy saucepan with the sugar and 2–4 tablespoons of water. Bring to the boil, then turn the heat down to low and simmer for about 10 minutes, or until the berries have burst. Mash a little with the back of a spoon or a fork, then cool and chill in the refrigerator. Adjust the flavour with a little more sugar, if you like.

Once the fruit has cooled thoroughly, whip the cream until thick, then fold it in. Serve chilled.

Serve sprinkled with granola or toasted nuts.

NUTRITION PROFILE (per portion)

5% protein, 23% fat, 66% carbohydrate, 6% fibre

VITAMINS AND MINERALS (percentage of RDA)

Vitamin C 29%, B1 9%, B2 12%, B5 8%, potassium 12%, calcium 7%, iron 5%, iodine 13%

HEALTH BENEFITS

Low calorie | strongly antioxidant | supports the immune system | may protect against cancer cell growth

Fresh Fruit Salad

Preparation time: 10 minutes | Calories per portion: 191

Serves 4

200g/7oz seasonal berries, rinsed and stalks removed

2 bananas, peeled and sliced

2 kiwi fruit, peeled and sliced

200g/7oz seedless red grapes, halved

50g/1¾oz/heaped ⅓ cup dry-roasted cashew nuts

50g/1¾oz dark/bittersweet chocolate, grated

a few sprigs of mint, finely chopped

Gently mix the fruits and berries together in a serving bowl. Sprinkle with the nuts, chocolate and mint leaves.

Serve with cream, ice cream or yogurt.

NUTRITION PROFILE (per portion)

7% protein, 35% fat, 54% carbohydrate, 4% fibre

VITAMINS AND MINERALS (percentage of RDA)

Vitamin C 29%, B1 11%, B6 17%, folate 9%, biotin 6%, potassium 21%, magnesium 10%, zinc 9%, selenium 7%

HEALTH BENEFITS

Low-calorie | strongly antioxidant | supports the immune system | benefits blood, hair and nails

Golden Berry Sorbet

You can make delicious sorbets by substituting any seasonal berries in place of the golden berries.

Preparation and cooking time: 15 minutes, plus cooling and freezing | Calories per portion: 162

Serves 4
200g/7oz/1 cup raw cane sugar
500g/1lb 2oz golden berries

Bring 100ml/3½fl oz/scant ½ cup water to the boil in a saucepan. Add the sugar and bring back to the boil for a few minutes longer, stirring all the time until the sugar has dissolved, then reduce the heat to a simmer and cook until the liquid has a syrupy consistency. Leave to cool thoroughly.

When cool, blend the golden berries to make a pulp and mix with the syrup. Stir well and freeze in a shallow, non-metal container for 4–6 hours. Take out of the freezer at least 15 minutes before serving.

NUTRITION PROFILE (per portion)
5% protein, 4% fat, 90% carbohydrate, 1% fibre

VITAMINS AND MINERALS (percentage of RDA)
Vitamin C 13%, B1 9%, B3 16%, iron 9%

HEALTH BENEFITS
Low calorie | may help reduce the effects of allergy-related conditions | benefits the skin and mucous membranes

Danish Raspberry Snitter

Snitter are traditional Danish pastries. Small, delicate and rectangular in shape, they are eaten as snacks or light meals, often accompanied by coffee or beer. They can be savoury as well as sweet, and different types may be served together. Raspberry snitter are the most popular of the sweet variety, and taste wonderful with a cup of good coffee.

Preparation and cooking time: 1 hour, plus chilling | Calories per snitter: 302

Serves 10
For the pastry dough
350g/12oz/2¾ cups plain/all-purpose flour
150g/5½oz cold vegetable margarine, diced
50g/1¾oz/heaped ⅓ cup icing/confectioners' sugar
1 egg, beaten

For the filling
200g/7oz raspberries
50g/1¾oz/¼ cup jam-making sugar
100g/3½oz/¾ cup icing/confectioners' sugar

Make the pastry dough by tipping the flour into a large bowl. Add the margarine by chopping it into the flour with a knife and spoon until it forms small lumps. Continue to rub the fat into the flour with your fingers until the mixture resembles fine breadcrumbs. Mix in the icing/confectioners' sugar and the egg to form a ball. Wrap the pastry dough in cling film/plastic wrap and place in the refrigerator for 30 minutes to chill.

Meanwhile, put the raspberries in a pan with the sugar and gradually bring to the boil. Turn the heat down to low, cover and leave the mixture to simmer gently for 15 minutes. Leave to cool.

Preheat the oven to 200°C/400°F/Gas 6. Place the chilled dough onto a piece of greaseproof/wax paper, a little larger than your baking sheet. Put another piece of greaseproof/wax paper on top of the dough and roll it out into an even, rectangular sheet, 5mm/¼in thick. Remove the top sheet of paper and transfer the other sheet with the rolled-out dough onto the baking sheet. Bake the pastry for 10 minutes, or until it turns golden brown. Remove the pastry from the oven and leave it to cool.

Make a simple icing by sifting the icing/confectioners' sugar into a bowl and then beating in 1–2 tablespoons of hot water until smooth. Cover half the cooked pastry with the raspberry filling and the other half with the icing. Cut the pastry in half and place the half with the icing carefully on top of the one covered in raspberry filling. Using a sharp knife, slice the cake into 10 rectangles, each about 5x10cm/2x4in, then serve.

NUTRITION PROFILE (per portion)
9% protein, 36% fat, 51% carbohydrate, 4% fibre

VITAMINS AND MINERALS (percentage of RDA)
Vitamin A 5%, D 8%, B1 7%, B6 6%, folate 6%, iron 5%, zinc 5%

HEALTH BENEFITS
An energy booster | mildly laxative

Strawberry Shortcake

Children love this tasty, cheerful-looking and remarkably easy-to-make snack, which contains the perfect summery combination of strawberries and cream within a scone-style sponge (or shortcake).

Preparation and cooking time: 1 hour, plus cooling | Calories per portion: 153

Serves 8

For the cake

250g/9oz/2 cups plain/all-purpose flour

2 tsp baking powder

75g/2½oz cold vegetable margarine, diced, plus extra for greasing

3 tbsp raw cane sugar

1 egg, beaten

4 tbsp soy or rice milk

½ tsp vanilla extract

½ tsp icing/confectioners' sugar, for dusting

For the strawberry filling

100ml/3½fl oz/scant ½ cup soy whipping cream or double/heavy cream

100ml/3½fl oz/scant ½ cup plain soy yogurt

350g/12oz strawberries, hulled and sliced (reserving 8 whole strawberries for decoration)

Preheat the oven to 220°C/425°F/Gas 7 and grease a large baking sheet. In a bowl, sift together the flour and baking powder. Add the margarine by chopping it into the flour with a knife and spoon until it forms small lumps. Continue to rub the fat into the flour with your fingers until the mixture resembles fine breadcrumbs. Stir in the raw cane sugar. Mix the egg with the milk and vanilla, then pour into the dry ingredients. Stir together gently, mixing in all the liquid to form a soft dough. Gently pat the dough into a smooth ball, place it on a floured surface and roll out to make a 20cm/8in diameter disc. Transfer to the prepared baking sheet and bake in the middle of the oven for 10–15 minutes, or until firm and golden on top. Leave to cool on a wire/cooling rack.

For the filling, whip the cream and gently fold in the yogurt. Then slice the shortcake in half horizontally with a large bread knife. Carefully lift off the top layer using a cake slice or spatula, and cut it into 8 equal wedges. Place the bottom layer on a cake tray and spread two-thirds of the whipped cream mixture over it. Cover this with a layer of strawberry slices. Carefully place the 8 shortcake wedges on top, dust with the icing/confectioners' sugar and spoon a dollop of filling on top of each wedge, along with a whole strawberry. Cut the lower layer into wedges as you serve the cake.

NUTRITION PROFILE (per portion)
11% protein, 38% fat, 47% carbohydrate, 4% fibre

VITAMINS AND MINERALS (percentage of RDA)
Vitamin A 7%, D 10%, C 26%, B1 10%, B3 8%, B6 9%, folate 10%, iron 7%, zinc 7%

HEALTH BENEFITS
Antioxidant | astringent and mildly diuretic | a gentle laxative

Blueberry Muffins

Adding blueberries to your muffins brings real health benefits to a delicious treat. The crumb topping gives a contrasting sweet and spicy crunch to the texture, and the whole berries provide wonderful bursts of colour and flavour.

Preparation and cooking time: 35 minutes | Calories per muffin: 275

Makes 12 muffins

200g/7oz/1½ cups plain/all-purpose flour

2 tsp baking powder

150g/5½oz/¾ cup raw cane sugar

½ tsp fine sea salt

6 tbsp corn oil

1 egg, lightly beaten

6 tbsp milk

150g/5½oz blueberries

For the crumb topping

100g/3½oz/½ cup raw cane sugar

50g/1¾oz/heaped ⅓ cup plain/
  all-purpose flour

60g/2¼oz vegetable margarine, diced

1 tsp ground cinnamon

Preheat the oven to 200°C/400°F/Gas 6. Line a 12-hole muffin pan with paper cases/liners. Sift the flour and baking powder into a bowl, then stir in the sugar and salt. In a separate bowl, combine the oil, egg and milk, then stir this into the flour mixture. Fold in the berries, then spoon the mixture evenly into the cases/liners.

To make the crumb topping, mix together the sugar, flour, margarine and cinnamon with a fork. Sprinkle this over the muffins and bake immediately for about 20 minutes until firm and golden. Leave the muffins to cool completely before serving.

NUTRITION PROFILE (per portion)
5% protein, 41% fat, 53% carbohydrate, 1% fibre

VITAMINS AND MINERALS (percentage of RDA)
Vitamin A 6%, D 9%, E 13%, B1 8%, iron 7%, calcium 6%

HEALTH BENEFITS
General tonic and source of antioxidants | benefits the microcirculation

Forest Berry Cake

A forest walk becomes even more enjoyable if you remember to take along a small basket (or any container) to fill with seasonal berries. Try this recipe with any combination of the following: raspberries, blackberries, boysenberries, loganberries, elderberries or strawberries.

Preparation and cooking time: 45 minutes | Calories per portion: 244

Serves 8

250g/9oz/2 cups plain/all-purpose flour

2 tsp baking powder

150g/5½oz/¾ cup raw cane sugar

½ tsp fine sea salt

100g/3½oz cold vegetable margarine, diced, plus extra for greasing

1 egg, beaten

250ml/9fl oz/1 cup apple juice

300g/10½oz mixed forest fruits (see above)

50g/1¾oz/⅓ cup walnuts and/or hazelnuts, chopped

Preheat the oven to 200°C/400°F/Gas 6. Grease and line a 23cm/9in round baking pan. Mix all the dry ingredients together in a bowl. Add the margarine by chopping it into the flour with a knife and spoon until it forms small lumps. Continue to rub in the fat and flour until the mixture resembles fine breadcrumbs. Mix in the egg and apple juice to make a soft dough, then gently stir in the berries and nuts.

Transfer to the prepared baking pan and bake for 30 minutes, or until a skewer inserted into the middle comes out clean. Leave to cool on a wire/cooling rack, then serve cut into slices.

NUTRITION PROFILE (per portion)
8% protein, 40% fat , 48% carbohydrate, 4% fibre

VITAMINS AND MINERALS (percentage of RDA)
Vitamin A 10%, D 15%, E 5%, C 18%, B1 12%, B3 9%, B5 7%, B6 12%, B12 5%, folate 12%, biotin 8%, potassium 9%, magnesium 10%, iron 10%, zinc 9%

HEALTH BENEFITS
Natural energy booster | good for heart, blood and nerves | useful in convalescence

Sweet Cherry Twirls

Preparation and cooking time: 30 minutes, plus rising | Calories per twirl: 213

Makes 10 twirls

For the dough

30g/1oz vegetable margarine, plus extra for greasing

150ml/5fl oz/⅔ cup soy or rice milk

50g/1¾oz fresh yeast

1 tbsp sugar

½ tsp fine sea salt

250g/9oz/2 cups plain/all-purpose flour

icing/confectioners' sugar, to sprinkle

For the filling

50g/1¾oz vegetable margarine, softened

3 tbsp raw cane sugar

1 tsp ground cinnamon

200g/7oz cherries, pitted and quartered

Heat the margarine gently with the milk until melted. Pour into a mixing bowl and leave until tepid, then sprinkle in the yeast and let it dissolve. Add the sugar, salt and enough flour to make a soft dough. Knead the dough to a smooth consistency, then leave to rise in a warm place for about 45 minutes until doubled in size.

Preheat the oven to 220°C/425°F/Gas 7 and grease a baking sheet. Roll out the dough into a long rectangle. Spread the margarine over it, then sprinkle with sugar, cinnamon and cherries. Roll up to make a long sausage, then cut the dough into 10 slices. Place each slice on its side on the baking sheet, securing the outer pastry ends underneath. Sprinkle the slices with icing/confectioner's sugar and bake for 10 minutes, or until golden. Cool on a wire/cooling rack.

NUTRITION PROFILE (per portion)
12% protein, 31% fat, 52% carbohydrate, 5% fibre

VITAMINS AND MINERALS (percentage of RDA)
Vitamin A 17%, E 14%, B1 30%, B2 22%, B3 25%, B5 14%, B6 24%, folate 78%, biotin 19%, potassium 18%, magnesium 20%, iron 18%, zinc 18%, copper 43%, manganese 81%

HEALTH BENEFITS
Good energy release | may improve sleep | strengthens eyes, skin, hair, nails, blood and bones | antioxidant | good healing properties

Fiery Inca Chocolate

Golden berries are also known as Inca or Aztec berries and come from the same part of the world as the cocoa bean. Cocoa butter is the fatty part of the cocoa bean and remains solid at room temperature, which makes it a useful ingredient in melt-in-your-mouth chocolates. The pinch of cayenne adds a kick of heat to the sweetness of the fruit and nut chocolate. Cocoa butter is available from good health food stores and on the internet.

Preparation time: 10 minutes, plus chilling | Calories per portion: 115

Makes 20 slices

200g/7oz cocoa butter, chopped

200g/7oz cocoa powder

200ml/7fl oz/scant 1 cup agave syrup
  or clear honey

50g/1¾oz/heaped ⅓ cup Brazil nuts,
  chopped

a pinch of cayenne pepper, to taste

100g/3½oz golden berries

Melt the cocoa butter in a heatproof bowl over a pan of simmering water. Take off the heat and stir in the cocoa powder, agave syrup, nuts and cayenne pepper.

Line a 23cm/9in square cake pan with kitchen foil and pour in the mixture. Allow the mixture to cool a little but not to solidify, then press the golden berries into the chocolate base in an even grid.

Chill in the refrigerator for about 30 minutes until solid. Remove from the pan and cut into 20 small slices.

NUTRITION PROFILE (per portion)
7% protein, 72% fat, 17% carbohydrate, 4% fibre

VITAMINS AND MINERALS (percentage of RDA)
Vitamin C 5%, potassium 5%, magnesium 10%, iron 6%, zinc 7%, selenium 7%

HEALTH BENEFITS
Soothing and comforting | benefits the heart and circulation | boosts metabolism | contains antioxidants that support the immune system

Berry and Nut Slices

Children love these raw power bars, and they make a perfect snack or travel food. They also taste delicious with a cup of after-dinner coffee! Once they have been cooled down, they hang together really well, but try to avoid leaving them in the sun, or in a bag next to a radiator, as they will lose their good texture if overheated. You can experiment with a variety of nuts and berries or other dried fruit, for example replacing jujube with dates, or goji with dried barberries or cranberries. Brazil nuts give a nice, neutral taste, hazelnuts go well with a dash of vanilla, and walnuts add a more 'grown-up' edge.

Preparation time: 10 minutes, plus chilling | Calories per portion: 166

Makes 20 slices

200g/7oz/scant 1⅔ cups cashew nuts

100g/3½oz/scant 1½ cups shredded fresh or desiccated/dried shredded coconut

150g/5½oz pitted jujube berries

1 tsp powdered açai berries

a pinch of fine sea salt

50g/1¾oz dried goji berries, plus extra for decoration

For the topping

100g/3½oz/heaped ¾ cup cashew nuts, plus extra for decoration

100g/3½oz/scant 1½ cups shredded fresh or desiccated/dried shredded coconut, plus extra for decoration

2 tbsp coconut oil

2 tbsp maple syrup

50g/1¾oz/⅓ cup dark/bittersweet chocolate chips, plus extra for decoration

1 tsp vanilla extract

To make the base, put the cashews, coconut, jujubes, açai powder and salt in a food processor and blend to a coarse, sticky consistency. Add the goji berries and blend for a few seconds longer. Line a dish, about 23cm/9in square, with greaseproof/wax paper, spread the mixture evenly onto it and press down to make a firm base.

Put all the topping ingredients in a blender. Add about 100ml/3½fl oz/scant ½ cup water and blend until smooth. Spread the topping over the base. Decorate

with a few more nuts, coconut, berries and chocolate drops and mark into
20 squares. Chill in the refrigerator for at least 30 minutes, or until solid, then
cut into squares and serve.

NUTRITION PROFILE (per portion)
10% protein, 71% fat, 18% carbohydrate, 2% fibre

VITAMINS AND MINERALS (percentage of RDA)
Vitamin E 6%, C 5%, B1 10%, B6 6%, folate 6%, potassium 9%, magnesium 13%,
iron 11%, zinc 10%, copper 37%, selenium 8%

HEALTH BENEFITS
Energy booster | antioxidant | rich in monounsaturated and omega oils | good for heart,
circulation and stress relief | may inhibit inflammation

PRESERVES AND
CONDIMENTS

Cloudberry Chutney

Cloudberries can be hard to find, but you can use this recipe to make chutney with most berries, especially those from the *Rubus* genus: blackberries, raspberries, boysenberries, or even mulberries. Whichever berries you choose, this is a chutney that goes well with a wide range of main courses, sandwiches and cheeses. Adjust the sweet/sour flavour by using more or less sugar or vinegar, according to the sweetness of the chosen berry.

Preparation and cooking time: 20 minutes | Calories per portion: 92

Makes about 300g/10½oz
50g/1¾oz/¼ cup raw cane sugar
1 red onion, finely chopped
4 juniper berries
2 tsp white wine vinegar
250g/9oz cloudberries
sea salt and freshly ground black pepper

Gently melt the sugar in a heavy pan over a low heat, stirring all the time. Add the onion and juniper berries and stir for a few minutes more until the onion is soft and coated in sugar. Stir in the vinegar and the cloudberries. Bring to the boil, then turn the heat down and simmer gently for about 10 minutes until the berries soften. Add salt and pepper to taste.

Pour into warm, sterilized jars (see page 182) and seal immediately. Store in a cool, dark place for up to 6 months.

NUTRITION PROFILE (per portion)
8% protein, 5% fat, 86% carbohydrate, 1% fibre

VITAMINS AND MINERALS (percentage of RDA)
Vitamin C 125%, B1 8%

HEALTH BENEFITS
High antioxidant content | naturally antibiotic | may help strengthen the immune system

Sloe Chutney

This is one of those recipes, like many in this section, for which it is difficult to give accurate timings and yield – so much depends on the ripeness of the fruit and how much liquid evaporates. As a variation, use damsons instead of sloes.

Preparation and cooking time: 2 hours | Calories per 100g/3½oz: 145

Makes about 1.5kg/3lb 5oz

1kg/2lb 4oz sloes, frozen or picked after
   first frost
2 cooking/baking apples, cored and
   chopped
2 white onions, chopped
250g/9oz/1¾ cups raisins
1 cinnamon stick
1 tsp whole cloves, crushed

1 tsp cayenne pepper
2.5cm/1in piece of root ginger, peeled
   and chopped
1 garlic clove, chopped
1 tsp salt
500g/1lb 2oz/2½ cups raw cane sugar
500ml/17fl oz/2 cups white wine vinegar

Place the sloes in a heavy saucepan, cover with water and bring to the boil, then simmer for about 20 minutes, or until soft. Pass the fruit through a sieve/fine-mesh strainer to remove the stones, then pour the purée back into the saucepan. Add the rest of the ingredients and bring to the boil again, stirring from time to time. Turn the heat to low and simmer, stirring occasionally, for about 1 hour until the mixture thickens. Remove the cinnamon stick and adjust the flavour with additional salt, sugar or vinegar, to taste.

Pour into warm, sterilized jars (see page 182) and seal immediately. Store in a cool, dark place for up to 6 months.

NUTRITION PROFILE (per portion)
3% protein, 3% fat, 88% carbohydrate, 6% fibre

VITAMINS AND MINERALS (percentage of RDA)
Vitamin C 40%, potassium 12%, iron 10%

HEALTH BENEFITS
High vitamin C | antiseptic and strong antioxidant

Raspberry and Apple Alliance

With their delicately coloured pink juice and finely balanced, sweetly acidic flavour, raspberries are perfect for making jam. Adding apples highlights the colour and provides pectin (see page 229) to yield a fine, glossy-pink, thick jam.

Preparation and cooking time: 40 minutes | Calories per 100g/3½oz: 218

Makes about 2kg/4lb 8oz
700g/1lb 9oz raspberries, rinsed
300g/10½oz cooking/baking apples, peeled, cored and finely chopped
2 tbsp lemon juice
1kg/2lb 4oz/5 cups light cane sugar

Put the raspberries in a heavy saucepan and top with the apples, lemon juice and sugar. Cover and leave to soften for 30 minutes, then bring to the boil slowly. Reduce the heat to cook gently for 5 minutes, stirring continuously. Remove from the heat and pour into warm, sterilized jars (see below). Seal immediately and store in a cool, dark place for up to 12 months.

Tip: Sterilize clean jars (along with their lids) in the oven at 130°C/250°F/Gas 1 for 20 minutes, making sure they are not touching. Carefully fill the jars with the hot preserve and seal while they are still hot. Do not fill hot jars with cold preserves or cold jars with hot preserves, or the jar may crack.

NUTRITION PROFILE (per portion)
2% protein, 0% fat, 96% carbohydrate, 2% fibre

VITAMINS AND MINERALS (percentage of RDA)
Vitamin C 17%

HEALTH BENEFITS
Antioxidant | helps the body fight inflammations and infections

Rowan Jelly

A tart jelly that goes well with game and strong cheeses. Freezing the berries for 24 hours before you use them makes the jelly less bitter.

Preparation and cooking time: 1 hour, plus overnight standing | Calories per 100g/3½oz: 152

Makes about 1kg/2lb 4oz
500g/1lb 2oz rowan berries, rinsed and stalks removed
500g/1lb 2oz unripe cooking/baking apples, cored and chopped
100g/3½oz/½ cup light cane sugar per 100ml/3½fl oz/scant ½ cup of juice
  (see method below)

Put the berries and the apples in a heavy saucepan with enough water to just cover them. Bring to the boil slowly over a medium-high heat, then turn the heat down to low and simmer for about 20 minutes, or until the berries disintegrate and release their juices. Pour the mixture into a muslin/cheesecloth bag set over a large bowl and leave it to filter through for 6–8 hours. Do not press the berries or the liquid will become cloudy.

Measure the amount of juice that has collected, then pour it back into the saucepan. Bring to the boil, then add the sugar slowly (100g/3½oz/½ cup for every 100ml/3½fl oz/scant ½ cup of juice). Stir well and simmer gently for about 10 minutes. Remove from the heat and pour into warm, sterilized jars (see page 182). Seal immediately and store in a cool, dark place for up to 12 months.

NUTRITION PROFILE (per portion)
2% protein, 3% fat, 93% carbohydrate, 2% fibre

VITAMINS AND MINERALS (percentage of RDA)
Vitamin A 16%, C 38%, iron 6%

HEALTH BENEFITS
A bitter astringent that stimulates fat digestion and relieves constipation

Cloudberry Preserve

Cloudberry is a delicious and delicate fruit that needs nothing but a little sugar to bring out its full flavour and preserve its goodness.

Preparation and cooking time: 30 minutes | Calories per 100g/3½oz: 145

Makes about 450g/1lb
300g/10½oz cloudberries, rinsed
150g/5½oz/¾ cup raw cane sugar

Rinse the cloudberries and put them in a saucepan with a splash of water – just enough to prevent them sticking. Add the sugar and heat through gently until it is dissolved, then bring slowly to the boil. Reduce the heat and simmer for 10 minutes. Pour into warm, sterilized jars (*see* page 182) and seal immediately. Store in a cool, dark place for up to 12 months.

NUTRITION PROFILE (per portion)
6% protein, 3% fat, 91% carbohydrate, 0% fibre

VITAMINS AND MINERALS (percentage of RDA)
Vitamin C 132%, iron 5%

HEALTH BENEFITS
Rich in vitamin C | promotes iron absorption | stimulates fat digestion and relieves constipation | general immune system stimulant

Rose Hip Jam

An excellent sweet and refreshingly different-tasting jam. You can also vary
the flavour combinations: try adding some vanilla, chopped apple, ginger
or almonds.

Preparation and cooking time: 45 minutes | Calories per 100ml/3½fl oz/
scant ½ cup: 236

Makes about 1l/35fl oz/4¼ cups
750g/1lb 10oz rose hips, rinsed, trimmed and deseeded (see page 153)
500g/1lb 2oz/2½ cups raw cane sugar
juice of 1 lemon

Chop the rose hips. Put them in a saucepan with 250ml/9fl oz/1 cup water and
bring to the boil. Turn the heat down to medium-low and leave to simmer for 10
minutes, then add the sugar and bring back to the boil, stirring from time to time for
a further 5 minutes. Add the lemon juice and heat through for 2 minutes. Pour into
warm, sterilized jars (see page 182) and seal immediately. Store in the refrigerator
for up to 12 months.

NUTRITION PROFILE (per portion)
2% protein, 2% fat, 91% carbohydrate, 5% fibre

VITAMINS AND MINERALS (percentage of RDA)
Vitamin A 10%, C 369%

HEALTH BENEFITS
Extremely high in vitamin C | encourages iron absorption and wound healing | increases
resistance to infections | may help to lower blood pressure and cholesterol levels

Countess Confiture

This is an old Danish recipe that first appeared in a book about preserves in 1939. Nobody knows where the name comes from, but this jam is rich and fine and fit for a countess! It is usually served with pancakes and waffles, but is also good served as a topping on open cheese sandwiches.

Preparation and cooking time: 45 minutes | Calories per 100ml/3½fl oz/scant ½ cup: 236

Makes about 1l/35fl oz/4¼ cups
500g/1lb 2oz elderberries, rinsed and stalks removed
500g/1lb 2oz cooking apples, peeled, cored and finely chopped
500g/1lb 2oz/2½ cups raw cane sugar
juice of 1 lemon

Mix the berries and apples in a saucepan, cover and heat gently for about 15 minutes until the fruit dissolves. Add the sugar, bring to the boil, stirring continuously, then reduce the heat and simmer for a further 10 minutes. Add the lemon juice and heat through. Pour into warm, sterilized jars (see page 182) and seal immediately. Store in a cool, dark place for up to 12 months.

NUTRITION PROFILE (per portion)
1% protein, 1% fat, 94% carbohydrate, 4% fibre

VITAMINS AND MINERALS (percentage of RDA)
Vitamin C 17%, B6 6%, iron 6%

HEALTH BENEFITS
A gentle laxative and natural aid to detox | warming and an astringent | can help control blood cholesterol levels

Berry Vinegar

Raspberries are a traditional and popular flavouring for vinegars, but boysenberries, cloudberries, dewberries, loganberries, mulberries, strawberries, cherries and most other berries will also give excellent results, allowing scope for endless experimentation. Use berry vinegars to add interesting colour and flavour to salad dressings, seasonings, court-bouillons, marinades and chutneys.

Preparation time: about 15 minutes, plus 1 week macerating | Calories per 100ml/3½fl oz/scant ½ cup: 32

Makes about 1.5l/52fl oz/6½ cups
1l/35floz/4¼ cups wine vinegar or apple cider vinegar
1kg/2lb 4oz berries, rinsed and stalks removed

Put the berries into a stoneware or glass jar (avoid using metal) and pour over the vinegar. Seal and leave to macerate for 1 week.

Strain the resulting flavoured vinegar into a container through a coffee filter or sieve/ strainer lined with muslin/cheesecloth, but do not press the berries. Pour into a sterilized bottle (see page 182) and seal immediately. Store in a cool, dark place for up to 6 months.

NUTRITION PROFILE (per portion)
9% protein, 4% fat, 86% carbohydrate, 1% fibre

VITAMINS AND MINERALS (percentage of RDA)
Vitamin C 20%, folate 8%, potassium 7%, magnesium 5%, iron 5%

HEALTH BENEFITS
Astringent | anti-inflammatory and antispasmodic | useful for treating coughs and colds, flu, arthritis, mouth ulcers and bleeding gums

Chilled Horseradish and Açai Sauce

Preparation time: 5 minutes, plus 1 hour chilling | Calories per portion: 79

Serves 4

4 tbsp fresh breadcrumbs

4 tbsp thick soy cream

4 tbsp grated fresh horseradish

1 tbsp açai berry powder

1 tbsp vinegar, or to taste

sea salt and raw cane sugar, to taste

Mix all the ingredients together in a small bowl. Adjust to taste with vinegar, salt and sugar. Chill in the refrigerator for 1 hour before serving.

Tip: You can replace the soy cream with almond, coconut, oat or dairy cream.

NUTRITION PROFILE (per portion)

12% protein, 26% fat, 54% carbohydrate, 8% fibre

VITAMINS AND MINERALS (percentage of RDA)

Vitamin C 28%, calcium 5%, iron 5%

HEALTH BENEFITS

Low calorie | strong immune booster | especially helpful in treatment of blocked sinuses and colds

Gooseberry Sauce

Preparation and cooking time: 40 minutes | Calories per portion: 87

Serves 4

1 tbsp grapeseed oil

1 shallot, finely chopped

250g/9oz gooseberries, trimmed

3 tbsp sugar

1 tbsp red wine vinegar

a pinch of ground cloves

sea salt and freshly ground black pepper

Heat the oil in a small saucepan, then add the shallot and gooseberries and stir-fry for 1 minute. Add 3 tablespoons water, the sugar, vinegar and cloves. Cover with a lid and cook gently over a medium heat for 20–25 minutes until the gooseberries are very soft. Season to taste and serve hot with game, duck, oily fish and nut roasts.

NUTRITION PROFILE (per portion)
4% protein, 37% fat, 53% carbohydrate, 6% fibre

VITAMINS AND MINERALS (percentage of RDA)
Vitamin C 18%, potassium 7%

HEALTH BENEFITS
Gently encourages immune defences against infection and cell degeneration

Red Berry Ketchup

This is a ketchup with a difference – tasty, spicy and healthy. You can use almost any combination of berries following this recipe, just adjust the sugar content accordingly. Serve it in place of regular commercial ketchup and add it to boost the flavour in marinades and dressings. Try it with burgers, shellfish, nut roast, poultry and game. Leave out the ginger and chilli for a milder, more child-friendly version.

Preparation and cooking time: 1 hour | Calories per 100ml/3½fl oz/scant ½ cup: 94

Makes 1l/35fl oz/4¼ cups

500g/1lb 2oz bearberries

500g/1lb 2oz cranberries or lingonberries

500g/1lb 2oz raspberries

500g/1lb 2oz tomatoes, chopped

2 red onions, chopped

2.5cm/1in piece of root ginger, peeled and chopped

1 small hot red chilli, chopped

1 tbsp paprika

1 tsp ground cinnamon

200ml/7fl oz/scant 1 cup white wine vinegar

500g/1lb 2oz/2½ cups raw cane sugar

sea salt and freshly ground black pepper

Strip all the berries from their stalks and rinse in cold water. Place them in a saucepan with the chopped tomatoes, onions, ginger, chilli, paprika and cinnamon. Add a little water, if necessary, to prevent any berries sticking to the bottom of the pan. Bring to the boil, then turn the heat down to low and simmer for 30 minutes.

Remove the pan from the heat and rub the mixture through a sieve/fine-mesh strainer with a wooden spoon. Discard the seeds and skins and return the remaining fruit pulp to a clean saucepan. Add the vinegar and sugar to the mixture and heat through, stirring from time to time, until the sugar is dissolved. Bring to the boil, then turn the heat down to low and simmer for approximately 5 minutes, stirring occasionally, until the sauce has a thick, ketchup-like consistency. Season with salt and pepper to taste, and adjust the flavour with a little more sugar or vinegar as necessary.

Pour into warm, sterilized bottles (see page 182) and seal immediately. Store in a cool, dark place for up to 12 months.

Tip: Try experimenting with other berries and spice combinations to produce a range of delicious ketchups.

NUTRITION PROFILE (per portion)
3% protein, 2% fat, 88% carbohydrate, 7% fibre

VITAMINS AND MINERALS (percentage of RDA)
Vitamin A 7%, C 20%

HEALTH BENEFITS
Warming | good for the heart and circulation | antioxidant content benefits immune system and strengthens resistance to infection

Pontack Sauce

This spicy elderberry sauce offers a traditional way of extending the elderberry season. Before the advent of freezers, each berry glut would provoke a flurry of pickling and preserving with sugar, spices and vinegar, and techniques for keeping nature's precious gifts were passed down through the generations. This not only allowed cooks to add interest to a restricted winter menu, but also provided means to help ward off the ailments that commonly accompanied the colder, darker months. This sauce is also known as 'elderberry ketchup', and makes a fine accompaniment to rich meals, and a delicious base for gravies. It dates back to a 17th-century British recipe named after 'Monsieur Pontack', the owner of 'London's first fashionable eating house', who was said to have invented it. Pontack sauce is famed for getting better the longer you store it as the flavours mature with age. A sealed jar of Pontack sauce can be kept for up to 7 years, but it can also be used immediately.

Preparation and cooking time: 1 hour | Calories per 100ml/3½fl oz/scant ½ cup: 161

Makes 1l/35fl oz/4¼ cups

1 tbsp olive oil

1 large onion, chopped

1.5kg/3lb 5oz elderberries, rinsed and stalks removed

1 tsp sea salt

500ml/17fl oz/2 cups malt vinegar

1 tbsp pickling spice

1kg/2lb 4oz/5 cups raw cane sugar

Heat the oil in a saucepan and cook the onion until soft. Stir in the rest of the ingredients and heat through gently until the sugar is dissolved. Bring to the boil, then reduce the heat to a gentle simmer and cook for about 45 minutes, or until the liquid has thickened. Strain and pour into warm, sterilized jars (see page 182) and seal immediately.

Tip: The taste matures the longer the sauce is stored. At least 2 months is recommended.

NUTRITION PROFILE (per portion)
3% protein, 4% fat, 89% carbohydrate, 5% fibre

VITAMINS AND MINERALS (percentage of RDA)
Vitamin C 16%, B6 9%, potassium 8%

HEALTH BENEFITS
Antiviral and antiseptic I helpful against colds and flu I promotes general immunity

DRINKS
AND TONICS

Rose Hip and Lemon Tonic

A strengthening, vitamin C-rich tonic that is easy to make and to take, to help prevent and treat allergies and infections.

Preparation time: 15 minutes, plus 1 week standing | Calories per 100ml/3½fl oz/ scant ½ cup (undiluted): 100

Makes about 1l/35fl oz/4¼ cups
500g/1lb 2oz rose hips, rinsed and kept whole (see page 153)
1 unwaxed lemon, washed and sliced, plus extra to serve
750ml/26fl oz/3¼ cups white wine
sparkling water, to dilute

Place the rose hips and lemon slices in a large glass jar. Add the wine, seal and store in the refrigerator. After a week, strain and serve diluted with sparkling water and a slice of lemon.

NUTRITION PROFILE (per portion)
3% protein, 1% fat, 82% carbohydrate, 14% fibre

VITAMINS AND MINERALS (percentage of RDA)
Vitamin A 20%, E 18%, C 204%

HEALTH BENEFITS
Extremely high in vitamin C | antibacterial and antioxidant | boosts resistance to infection | enhances iron absorption | helps lower blood fat levels

Rowan and Sea-Buckthorn Syrup

Also called 'Scandinavian lemons', rowan and sea-buckthorn berries have long been used in Nordic countries as a source of vitamin C. As a bonus, they also contain high levels of vitamin A. Rapadura is unbleached, unrefined raw cane sugar, which gives a distinctive caramel taste to these slightly bitter, acidic berries.

Preparation and cooking time: 50 minutes, plus standing | Calories per 100ml/3½fl oz/scant ½ cup (undiluted): 148

Makes about 1l/35fl oz/4¼ cups

500g/1lb 2oz rowan berries, rinsed and stalks removed

500g/1lb 2oz sea-buckthorn berries, rinsed

500g/1lb 2oz/2½ cups rapadura or raw cane sugar

juice of 1 lemon

Put the berries and 500ml/17fl oz/2 cups water in a saucepan. Bring to the boil, reduce the heat to low and simmer for 10 minutes. Mash the berries and strain through a filter, letting the berry juice drip down into another pan for about 30 minutes. Gradually bring the juice to the boil while adding the sugar, stirring continuously until the sugar is dissolved. Add the lemon juice and leave the syrup to cool for 5 minutes. Pour into warm sterilized bottles (see page 182), seal immediately and store in a cool, dark place for up to 6 months. Serve diluted with water.

Tip: Both berry varieties benefit from being frozen before use; rowans lose some of their bitterness and sea-buckthorn berries are easier to pick off their thorny branches.

NUTRITION PROFILE (per portion)
2% protein, 14% fat, 84% carbohydrate, 0% fibre

VITAMINS AND MINERALS (percentage of RDA)
Vitamin A 18%, C 116%, B2 26%, B3 106%, B6 20%, potassium 13%, iron 61%

HEALTH BENEFITS
Antioxidant, antibiotic and an astringent | aids fat digestion | promotes efficient energy metabolism

Sweet Berry Cough Mixture

Make this cough remedy in the autumn while the berries are fresh, then keep it in the refrigerator ready to soothe coughs and colds when winter comes. Make more using frozen berries if you run out. Take one or two teaspoonfuls as needed.

Preparation and cooking time: 45 minutes, plus straining | Calories per 100ml/3½fl oz/scant ½ cup: 109

Makes about 750ml/26fl oz/3¼ cups

200g/7oz blackcurrants rinsed, and stalks removed

200g/7oz blackberries, rinsed

200g/7oz elderberries, rinsed and stalks removed

2 tbsp red wine vinegar

200ml/7fl oz/scant 1 cup clear honey or syrup

1 tbsp liquorice powder

5 star anise

Put the berries in a heavy saucepan. Add the vinegar and 1 tablespoon of water and bring to the boil, stirring from time to time. Cover and leave to simmer gently for 15 minutes until the berries have disintegrated and released their juices.

Strain the pulp into a container through a filter or sieve/strainer lined with muslin/cheesecloth and pour the juice back into the pan. Add the honey, liquorice powder and star anise, then bring the mixture back to the boil, stirring occasionally. Turn the heat down to low and leave to simmer for 5 minutes (but be careful not to let it boil over, it is very sticky to clean up). Strain again and immediately pour into a warm, sterilized bottle (see page 182). Seal and leave to cool, shaking from time to time. Store in the refrigerator for up to 6 months.

NUTRITION PROFILE (per portion)
5% protein, 5% fat, 82% carbohydrate, 8% fibre

VITAMINS AND MINERALS (percentage of RDA)
Vitamin C 68%, potassium 12%, iron 20%

HEALTH BENEFITS
Rich in vitamin C and iron | healing and soothing | antiviral, antibacterial and gentle laxative

Juniper Tincture

Unsurprisingly, juniper tincture tastes like gin and is both warming and stimulating. Herbalists use it as a diuretic, and to calm and improve digestion. Take ½–1 teaspoon of the tincture three times a day to ease kidney and bladder complaints, and treat aching muscles due to excess lactic acid.

WARNING
Do not use internally for more than 2 weeks at a time. Avoid during pregnancy.

Macerating time: 2 weeks | Calories per 100ml/3½fl oz/scant ½ cup: 148

Makes about 700ml/24fl oz/3 cups
300g/10½oz juniper berries
700ml/24fl oz/3 cups whisky, brandy or vodka (40% alcohol)

Put the berries into a 1l/35fl oz/4¼ cups glass jar. Add the alcohol and close the lid tightly. Keep at room temperature for 2 weeks and shake well each morning and evening. Strain through a filter or sieve/strainer lined with muslin/cheesecloth and decant into sterilized dark bottles (see page 182).

Tip: You can also use this basic recipe to make hawthorn tincture, which is a traditional remedy for high blood pressure and for strengthening the heart and circulation.

NUTRITION PROFILE (per portion)
Negligible

VITAMINS AND MINERALS (percentage of RDA)
Negligible

HEALTH BENEFITS
Antioxidant | anti-inflammatory | improves digestion | treats kidney and bladder complaints | relieves aching joints and muscles

Sea-Buckthorn, Orange and Carrot Slush

This bright orange slush is a potent immune-stimulating, vitamin and mineral boost. It is an excellent remedy for healing and repairing, and helps to combat infections and ease chronic diseases.

Preparation time: 5 minutes | Calories per serving: 230

Serves 1

50g/1¾oz sea-buckthorn berries, rinsed

2 oranges, peeled, pith and pips removed

2 carrots, finely chopped

1cm/½in piece of root ginger, peeled and chopped

2 ice cubes

Press the berries through a sieve/fine-mesh strainer to remove the seeds. Blend the berry pulp together with the rest of the ingredients and serve immediately.

NUTRITION PROFILE (per portion)
10% protein, 16% fat, 62% carbohydrate, 12% fibre

VITAMINS AND MINERALS (percentage of RDA)
Vitamin A 162%, E 26%, C 396%, B1 38%, B2 65%, B3 228%, B5 32%, B6 74%, B12 108%, folate 65%, potassium 58%, calcium 34%, magnesium 16%, iron 115%, zinc 13%, selenium 6%

HEALTH BENEFITS
Extremely high in vitamins | boosts immunity | helps combat infections

Autumn Gold Smoothie

If you are armed with a good blender, this golden smoothie is super-easy to prepare and packed with nutrients. Filling and easily digestible, it makes an energy-boosting snack at any time of day.

Preparation time: 5 minutes | Calories per serving: 226

Serves 2

10 golden berries

1 tbsp dried goji berries

1 tbsp cashew nuts

1 banana, peeled

¼ pineapple, peeled, cored and roughly chopped

½ mango, peeled and pitted

1 large date, pitted

4 ice cubes

Blend all the ingredients together until smooth and serve immediately.

NUTRITION PROFILE (per portion)
9% protein, 18% fat, 69% carbohydrate, 4% fibre

VITAMINS AND MINERALS (percentage of RDA)
Vitamin A 13%, E 10%, C 69%, B1 23%, B2 10%, B3 17%, B5 10%, B6 28%, folate 10%, biotin 5%, potassium 31%, calcium 6%, magnesium 18%, iron 18%, zinc 8%, selenium 5%

HEALTH BENEFITS
Boosts immunity | benefits digestion | promotes efficient release of energy

Açai Energy Shake

A vibrant and nourishing energy lift to pick you up after a long day, or to help you wake up in the morning.

Preparation time: 5 minutes | Calories per serving: 164

Serves 2

1 tbsp açai pulp, dried or frozen

1 banana, peeled

100g/3½oz strawberries, hulled

100g/3½oz blueberries

200ml/7fl oz/scant 1 cup almond milk

2 tsp maple syrup

1–2 drops vanilla extract (optional)

Blend all the ingredients until smooth. Add a little water to adjust the consistency, if preferred. Pour into glasses and serve immediately.

Tip: You can use fresh or frozen berries.

NUTRITION PROFILE (per portion)
8% protein, 9% fat, 75% carbohydrate, 8% fibre

VITAMINS AND MINERALS (percentage of RDA)
Vitamin A 32%, E 79%, C 122%, B1 10%, B2 9%, B3 11%, B5 14%, B6 29%, folate 20%, biotin 7%, potassium 33%, calcium 28%, magnesium 14%, iron 11%, zinc 9%, iodine 11%

HEALTH BENEFITS
Packed with essential nutrients and antioxidants | increases energy and stamina | enhances immunity | protects against infection

Chocolate Cherry Shake

Preparation time: 5 minutes | Calories per serving: 236

Serves 2

50g/1¾oz dark/bittersweet chocolate, broken into pieces

200g/7oz fresh or frozen cherries, pitted

200ml/7fl oz/scant 1 cup almond milk

1 tbsp açai pulp, dried or frozen

¼ tsp chilli powder

ice cubes (optional)

Blend all the ingredients to a smooth, creamy consistency. Add ice cubes if you prefer a thinner consistency.

NUTRIENT BALANCE (per portion)
8% protein, 31% fat, 55% carbohydrate, 6% fibre

VITAMINS AND MINERALS (percentage of RDA)
Vitamin A 20%, E 38%, C 13%, potassium 15%, calcium 14%, magnesium 9%, iron 8%, zinc 4%, selenium 4%

HEALTH BENEFITS
A calming energy booster | good for mind, body and spirit | antioxidant | benefits eyes, skin and immune system | helps protect against heart disease and cancer

Blue-Berry Smoothie

This thick, cool and creamy smoothie is a perfect energy booster at any time of day and makes a quick and easy substitute for a meal. You can replace the honeyberries with blackberries, boysenberries, red grapes, loganberries or mulberries, and substitute dates for the jujube berries.

Preparation time: 5 minutes | Calories per serving: 73

Serves 2
100g/3½oz blueberries
100g/3½oz honeyberries
5 pitted jujube berries
100ml/3½fl oz/scant ½ cup almond milk
ice cubes, to taste

Blend all the ingredients together until smooth and serve immediately.

NUTRITION PROFILE (per portion)
16% protein, 35% fat, 45% carbohydrate, 4% fibre

VITAMINS AND MINERALS (percentage of RDA)
Vitamin A 8%, E 20%, C 14%, B1 11%, B2 14%, potassium 15%, calcium 14%, magnesium 6%, iron 8%, copper 16%

HEALTH BENEFITS
Energy booster | increases metabolism | benefits circulation and digestion | rich in anti-oxidants | helps lower cholesterol | good for the heart and circulation

Blackcurrant, Banana and Cashew Shake

Blackcurrants add colour and edge to this rich energy drink.

Preparation time: 5 minutes | Calories per serving: 168

Serves 2

200ml/7fl oz/scant 1 cup soy milk

100g/3½oz blackcurrants, rinsed and stalks removed

25g/1oz/scant ¼ cup cashew nuts, or 2 tbsp cashew butter

1 banana, peeled

1 tsp clear honey (optional)

ice cubes, to serve

Blend all the ingredients, except the honey, until smooth. Add a little honey to sweeten, if you like, and serve with ice.

NUTRITION PROFILE (per portion)
16% protein, 41% fat, 39% carbohydrate, 4% fibre

VITAMINS AND MINERALS (percentage of RDA)
Vitamin E 12%, C 124%, B1 16%, B2 23%, B5 8%, B6 21%, folate 16%, biotin 8%, potassium 28%, calcium 8%, magnesium 19%, iron 13%, zinc 11%, selenium 7%

HEALTH BENEFITS
Vitamin booster | helps lower cholesterol and LDL fat levels | keeps skin, hair, glands, nerves, mucous membranes, blood cells and bone marrow healthy

Spring Dawn

Preparation time: 5 minutes | Calories per serving: 314

Serves 2

2 persimmons, stalks removed, quartered

1 orange, peeled, pith and pips removed, sliced

1 banana, peeled

200ml/7fl oz/scant 1 cup coconut milk

a pinch of ground cinnamon

ice cubes (optional)

Blend all the ingredients until smooth. Add a little water or ice for a thinner consistency, if you like.

NUTRITION PROFILE (per portion)
6% protein, 28% fat, 60% carbohydrate, 7% fibre

VITAMINS AND MINERALS (percentage of RDA)
Vitamin A 23%, E 8%, C 142%, B1 22%, B2 13%, B3 12%, B5 16%, B6 37%, folate 40%, biotin 8%, potassium 45%, calcium 16%, magnesium 22%, iron 22%, zinc 10%, selenium 6%

HEALTH BENEFITS
Nutritious | high energy | blood sugar stabilizer | good for skin, hair and nails | benefits bones and blood vessels

Summer Sun

Low in calories yet filling, this drink is almost a meal in itself. It can be used as part of a slimming regime and in other situations where calorie control is important, such as diabetes. This recipe works equally well with raspberries, mulberries, dewberries or loganberries.

Preparation time: 5 minutes | Calories per serving: 199

Serves 2
200g/7oz cherries, pitted
50g/1¾oz boysenberries
1 banana, peeled
200ml/7fl oz/scant 1 cup soy yogurt
¼ tsp vanilla extract
maple syrup, to taste
ice cubes (optional)

Blend the cherries, berries, banana, yogurt and vanilla until smooth. Add maple syrup to taste, and adjust the consistency by adding a few ice cubes, if you like.

NUTRITION PROFILE (per portion)
15% protein, 20% fat, 60% carbohydrate, 5% fibre

VITAMINS AND MINERALS (percentage of RDA)
Vitamin A 4%, E 17%, C 22%, B5 9%, B6 16%, folate 14%, biotin 4%, potassium 23%, magnesium 9%, iron 4%

HEALTH BENEFITS
Low in calories but high in the feeling-full factor | brain-power boost

Winter Wonder

Preparation time: 5 minutes | Calories per serving: 257

Serves 2

2 kiwi fruit, peeled and quartered

20 seedless red grapes

1 thick slice of fresh coconut flesh, chopped

150ml/5fl oz/⅔ cup dairy-free vanilla ice cream

Blend all the ingredients together until smooth and serve immediately.

NUTRITION PROFILE (per portion)
6% protein, 42% fat, 47% carbohydrate, 3% fibre

VITAMINS AND MINERALS (percentage of RDA)
Vitamin C 48%, B1 13%, B2 16%, B6 11%, B12 21%, biotin 5%, potassium 23%, calcium 10%, magnesium 7%, selenium 4%

HEALTH BENEFITS
Quick antioxidant energy lift that can help in the prevention of colds and flu

Gooseberry and Pineapple Smoothie

Gooseberries and pineapple share the same sweet-sharp qualities, and complement each other especially well when sweetened with banana and ice cream.

Preparation time: 5 minutes | Calories per serving: 190

Serves 2

100g/3½oz gooseberries, trimmed

2 thick slices of pineapple, peeled

1 banana, peeled

100ml/3½fl oz/scant ½ cup dairy-free vanilla ice cream

1 tbsp maple syrup

ice cubes (optional)

Blend all the ingredients, except the maple syrup and ice cubes, to make a creamy consistency. Add maple syrup to taste and ice cubes to give a thinner consistency, if you like. Serve immediately.

NUTRITION PROFILE (per portion)
6% protein, 21% fat, 69% carbohydrate, 4% fibre

VITAMINS AND MINERALS (percentage of RDA)
Vitamin C 36%, B1 15%, B2 14%, B5 11%, B6 16%, folate 10, biotin 6%, potassium 25%, calcium 8%, magnesium 8%, iron 5%

HEALTH BENEFITS
Increases immune defence | stimulates digestion | good for heart and circulation | aids tissue repair

Summer Berry Lemonade

For the best, full summer flavour, use whichever seasonal berries you can find, fresh or frozen. Try a range of berry combinations including blackberry, boysenberry, cloudberry, dewberry, loganberry, mulberry, raspberry, red- and blackcurrant or strawberry.

Preparation time: 20 minutes, plus chilling | Calories per serving: 127

Serves 2

200g/7oz/1 cup golden caster/granulated sugar

peel from 1 unwaxed lemon

100g/3½oz mixed summer berries, rinsed and stalks removed

juice of 8 lemons

To serve

100g/3½oz frozen cherries

ice cubes, still or sparkling water, to taste

Put 500ml/17fl oz/2 cups water, the sugar and lemon peel in a saucepan and bring to the boil. Stir occasionally to help the sugar dissolve, then turn the heat down to low, cover and simmer for a few more minutes until the mixture has become a clear and glossy syrup. Discard the lemon peel and set the syrup aside.

Blend the summer berries and press the pulp through a sieve/fine-mesh strainer over a bowl to remove the seeds. Add the syrup and lemon juice to the sieved berry pulp, together with a further 500ml/17fl oz/2 cups water. Cover and chill in the refrigerator for about 30 minutes. Serve with the frozen cherries, ice cubes and still or sparkling water, according to taste.

NUTRITION PROFILE (per portion)
2% protein l0% fat, 95% carbohydrate, 3% fibre

VITAMINS AND MINERALS (percentage of RDA)
Vitamin C 13%, potassium 4%, calcium 3%, iron 4%

HEALTH BENEFITS
Light and refreshing | good for summer colds and allergies

Elderberry Cordial

This basic cordial recipe can be used with a variety of other berries, including redcurrant, blackcurrant, cranberry, blackberry, strawberry, cherry or even sloes.

Preparation time: 45 minutes | Calories per 100ml/3½fl oz/scant ½ cup: 98

Makes about 1l/35fl oz/4¼ cups
1kg/2lb 4oz elderberries, rinsed and stalks removed
2 cooking/baking apples, chopped and cored
400g/14oz/2 cups raw cane sugar or rapadura sugar
juice of 1 lemon
1 tsp citric acid
still or sparkling water, to serve

Place the elderberries in a heavy saucepan with 500ml/17fl oz/2 cups water and the apples. Bring gently to the boil and heat through until the berries burst. Strain through a filter or a sieve/strainer lined with a piece of muslin/cheesecloth into a saucepan. Add the sugar, lemon juice and citric acid to the saucepan with the strained elderberry juice. Bring to the boil and heat through to let the sugar dissolve. Skim off any froth and pour into warm, sterilized bottles (see page 182). Seal and store in a cool, dark place for up to 6 months. Drink the cordial diluted with still or sparkling water, or with hot water for a non-alcoholic alternative to mulled wine.

NUTRITION PROFILE (per portion)
2% protein, 2% fat, 89% carbohydrate, 7% fibre

VITAMINS AND MINERALS (percentage of RDA)
Vitamin C 17%, B6 8%, potassium 7%, iron 6%

HEALTH BENEFITS
A traditional winter cold remedy with potent antiviral properties | boosts immunity | useful in the management of arthritis and skin infections

Raw Cranberry and Grape Juice

Preparation time: 5 minutes | Calories per serving: 98

Serves 2

100g/3½oz fresh cranberries

200g/7oz seedless red grapes

1 tbsp maple syrup (optional)

still or sparkling water, to serve

Blend or juice the berries and grapes. Sweeten with maple syrup, if you like, and serve diluted with still or sparkling water.

NUTRITION PROFILE (per portion)

2% protein, 2% fat, 90% carbohydrate, 6% fibre

VITAMINS AND MINERALS (percentage of RDA)

Vitamin C 24%, B1 12%, B6 19%, potassium 27%, iron 11%, zinc 10%

HEALTH BENEFITS

A proven remedy for the relief of cystitis | rich in antioxidants | benefits body cells

Autumn Berry Fizz

Preparation time: 5 minutes | Calories per serving: 102

Serves 2
300g/10½oz raspberries
100g/3½oz blackcurrants, rinsed and stalks removed
sparkling apple juice, to taste
ice cubes, to serve

Blend or juice the raspberries and blackcurrants. Pour into two tall glasses and top up with the apple juice and ice. Serve immediately.

NUTRITION PROFILE (per portion)
10% protein, 4% fat, 61% carbohydrate, 25% fibre

VITAMINS AND MINERALS (percentage of RDA)
Vitamin E 10%, C 194%, B5 10%, B6 10%, folate 26%, biotin 9%, potassium 25%, calcium 9%, magnesium 11%, iron 13%, zinc 6%

HEALTH BENEFITS
Low calorie | vitamin C booster | good for treating and preventing colds and flu

Fruit of the Vine

Preparation time: 5 minutes | Calories per serving: 154

Serves 2

4 kiwi fruit, peeled and quartered, a few slices reserved for decoration

250g/9oz seedless red grapes

1 tsp lemon juice

ice cubes, to serve

sparkling water, to serve

Blend or juice the kiwi fruit and grapes with the lemon juice. Pour into two large wine glasses, then fill up with ice and sparkling water. Decorate with the reserved kiwi slices and serve.

NUTRITION PROFILE (per portion)
5% protein, 4% fat, 84% carbohydrate, 7% fibre

VITAMINS AND MINERALS (percentage of RDA)
Vitamin C 95%, B6 22%, potassium 31%, calcium 6%, magnesium 7%, iron 6%

HEALTH BENEFITS
Helps to reduce blood cholesterol levels and the risk of blood clots | may help in the prevention and treatment of high blood pressure

Dewberry Sparkle

If dewberries are hard to find, blackberries, loganberries or raspberries make good substitutes.

Preparation time: 10 minutes | Calories per serving: 141

Serves 2
200g/7oz dewberries
3 carrots, scrubbed
1 apple, cored and quartered
1 pear, cored and quartered
sparkling water, to serve
ice cubes (optional)

Juice the berries, carrots, apple and pear, or blend them with a little water. Pour the juice into two glasses, add sparkling water and ice, if you like, and serve.

NUTRITION PROFILE (per portion)
7% protein, 5% fat, 74% carbohydrate, 14% fibre

VITAMINS AND MINERALS (percentage of RDA)
Vitamin A 197%, E 16%, C 19%, B1 15%, B2 13%, B6 13%, folate 11%, potassium 17%

HEALTH BENEFITS
Gives a powerful vitamin A and carotenoid boost | benefits the skin, eyes and reproductive system | helps maintain the immune system

Aronia Fruit Punch

Preparation time: 10 minutes | Calories per serving: 132

Serves 2

100g/3½oz aronia berries, a few reserved for decoration

50g/1¾oz frozen sea-buckthorn berries

100g/3½oz cherries, pitted

100g/3½oz strawberries, hulled

1 sweet red apple, cored and cubed

ice cubes, to serve

sparkling red grape juice, to taste

maple syrup (optional)

Blend or juice the berries and the apple. Pour the juice into two cocktail glasses, add the reserved whole berries and top up with ice cubes and sparkling red grape juice. Sweeten with maple syrup, if you like, and serve immediately.

NUTRITION PROFILE (per portion)
6% protein, 15% fat, 67% carbohydrate, 12% fibre

VITAMINS AND MINERALS (percentage of RDA)
Vitamin A 6%, E 16%, C 156%, B2 29%, B3 110%, B5 9%, B6 26%, folate 16%, potassium 25%, calcium 10%, magnesium 8%, iron 62%, zinc 7%

HEALTH BENEFITS
Immune boosting | useful in the treatment of acute infections, especially of the urinary tract | may relieve stomach problems and chronic inflammations

In the Pink

Preparation time: 5 minutes | Calories per serving: 150

Serves 2

50g/1¾oz blueberries

50g/1¾oz blackberries

50g/1¾oz strawberries

100g/3½oz raspberries

100g/3½oz cherries, pitted

ice cubes, to serve

Rinse and trim all the berries, then blend together and serve with ice.

NUTRITION PROFILE (per portion)
9% protein, 4% fat, 67% carbohydrate, 19% fibre

VITAMINS AND MINERALS (percentage of RDA)
Vitamin E 16%, C 122%, B1 9%, B2 10%, B3 9%, B5 15%, B6 14%, folate 34%, biotin 7%, potassium 29%, calcium 9%, magnesium 13%, iron 12%, zinc 7%

HEALTH BENEFITS
Powerful antioxidant repair for all body cells

Loganberry and Orange Juice

This refreshing and health-giving juice works equally well with a half-and-half mixture of blackberries and raspberries, if you can't find any loganberries.

Preparation time: 15 minutes | Calories per serving: 131

Serves 1

200g/7oz loganberries

2 oranges, halved and juiced

maple syrup (optional)

ice cubes, to serve

slice of lemon, to serve

Mash the berries through a sieve/fine-mesh strainer into a bowl and discard the seeds. Add the orange juice to the berry juice in the bowl. Sweeten the juice with maple syrup, if you like. Serve with ice cubes and a slice of lemon.

NUTRITION PROFILE (per portion)

9% protein, 0% fat, 76% carbohydrate, 15% fibre

VITAMINS AND MINERALS (percentage of RDA)

Vitamin E 10%, C 154%, B1 14%, B2 9%, B3 8%, B5 10%, B6 14%, folate 48%, biotin 10%, potassium 37%, calcium 12%, magnesium 17%, iron 24%, zinc 12%

HEALTH BENEFITS

High vitamin C content | promotes tissue healing | stimulates the immune system | helps maintain blood and nerve cells

Rowan, Apple and Carrot Juice

Rowan berries become sweeter when frozen. Pick them before the first frosts, then rinse, dry and store in the freezer. This is best made with a juicer.

Preparation time: 5 minutes | Calories per serving: 109

Serves 2
50g/1¾oz frozen rowan berries
1 sweet apple, quartered and cored
5 carrots, scrubbed
clear honey (optional)
ice cubes, to serve

Blend or juice the berries, apple and carrots. Sweeten the juice with honey, if you like, and serve with ice.

NUTRITION PROFILE (per portion)
6% protein, 10% fat, 73% carbohydrate, 11% fibre

VITAMINS AND MINERALS (percentage of RDA)
Vitamin A 215%, E 8%, C 40%, B1 6%, B5 5%, B6 8%, folate 19%, potassium 21%, calcium 7%, magnesium 5%, iron 7%

HEALTH BENEFITS
Antioxidant with high vitamin A and carotenoids | benefits blood, joints and respiratory system | promotes steady blood sugar levels

Mulberry Wine

This is the easy way to make a dessert wine without knowing anything about viticulture, and it has a great taste and even improves with age. Mulberries do not ripen at the same time, even on the same tree. Pick them every day as they become ripe and store them in the freezer until you need them.

Preparation and cooking time: 30 minutes | Maturing time: 6 months | Calories per 100ml/3½fl oz/scant ½ cup: 152

Makes about 1.6l/56fl oz/6½ cups

2 kg/4lb 8oz mulberries

300g/10½oz/1½ cups raw cane sugar

300ml/10½fl oz/1¼ cups brandy

Place the mulberries in a saucepan with 300ml/10½fl oz/1¼ cups water. Bring to the boil over a medium heat, then turn the heat down to low and simmer until the berries soften and release their juice. This should take 5–10 minutes. Strain through a sieve/strainer lined with muslin/cheesecloth. You should end up with about 1l/35fl oz/4¼ cups of juice. Pour this juice into a jar, add the sugar, cover with a plate, cool and leave in a cold place for 3 days, stirring and skimming off any froth every day.

Leave for another 5 days, stirring every day. Skim off the froth again. Add the brandy, then decant into an airtight container, leaving any sediment behind, and seal.

After another 2 days, decant into a sterilized bottle, again leaving any sediment behind. Cork and seal. Leave for 6 months before drinking.

NUTRITION PROFILE (per portion)
6% protein, 0% fat, 91% carbohydrate, 3% fibre

VITAMINS AND MINERALS (percentage of RDA)
Vitamin C 16%, folate 11%, potassium 9%, iron 9%

HEALTH BENEFITS
A traditional cold remedy | packed with antioxidant anthocyanins | helps lower blood cholesterol levels | may also protect against nerve cell degeneration

Crème de Cassis

A deliciously sweet and syrupy French liqueur made from fresh blackcurrants (*cassis*), this is traditionally served in small glasses as an apéritif with ice and water. It is also an essential ingredient in popular cocktails such as Kir Royale.

Preparation and cooking time: 25 minutes, plus standing | Maturing time: minimum 3 months | Calories per 100ml/3½fl oz/scant ½ cup: 286

Makes about 2l/70fl oz/8½ cups

1kg/2lb 4oz blackcurrants, rinsed and stalks removed

1l/35fl oz/4¼ cups 40% eau-de-vie (or vodka or brandy) and an extra 250ml/9fl oz/1 cup (see method below)

1kg/2lb 4oz/5 cups caster/granulated sugar per 1l/35fl oz/4¼ cups of filtered liquid (see method below)

Place the blackcurrants in a sterilized glass jar or bottle and fill right to the top with your chosen alcohol. Put the lid on tightly and leave in a cool dark place for 3 months.

Pour the berry/alcohol mix into a large bowl or pan. Mash the berries with a potato masher, then filter through a fine sieve/strainer and collect the liquor in a large saucepan, which may take several hours. Measure the amount: for every 1l/35fl oz/4¼ cups of filtered liquid, add 1kg/2lb 4oz of sugar and another 250ml/9fl oz/1 cup of eau-de-vie. Heat through, stirring continuously, until the sugar is completely dissolved and it looks syrupy, skimming off any froth from the surface. Be careful not to heat for too long or you'll end up with jelly instead of liqueur. Pour into warm sterilized bottles (see page 182) while hot and seal firmly. Store in a cool, dark place. You could drink it immediately but the longer you keep it, the better it gets.

NUTRITION PROFILE (per portion)
1% protein, 0% fat, 98% carbohydrate, 1% fibre

VITAMINS AND MINERALS (percentage of RDA)
Vitamin C 83%, potassium 7%, iron 5%

HEALTH BENEFITS
Stimulates digestion | good remedy for coughs and colds | benefits heart and circulation

Sloe Gin

Sloe gin has a wonderful red colour and a delicious, sweet, aromatic almond-like flavour with a hint of resin, which increases with age. The sugar is needed to extract the full flavour from the berries. Try adding a few cloves and a stick of cinnamon to make a spicier blend.

Maturing time: minimum 9 weeks | Calories per 100ml/3½fl oz/scant ½ cup: 231

Makes about 1.5l/52fl oz/6 cups
500g/1lb 2oz sloes, rinsed
250g/9oz/1¼ cups caster/granulated sugar
1l/35fl oz/4 cups gin

Prick through the sloes' skins with a sterilized skewer or needle. Put the pierced sloes in a large sterilized bottle or glass jar (see page 182). Add the sugar and the gin, then seal the bottle firmly and give it a good shake. Store in a cool, dark place and shake every day for a week, then every week for 2 months, by which time it will be dark red and ready to drink, but the longer you keep it, the better it gets.

NUTRITION PROFILE (per portion)
2% protein, 3% fat, 94% carbohydrate, 1% fibre

VITAMINS AND MINERALS (percentage of RDA)
Vitamin C 29%, iron 4%

HEALTH BENEFITS
A traditional flu remedy | effective against bacterial infections | aids digestion

Wild Damson Brandy

Damson brandy is better known as *Slivovitz*, a favourite drink in the Balkan and Slavic countries. It is thought to have first been produced in the 14th century by Bulgarian monks at the Troyan Monastery, which still exists, and damsons are still celebrated in this region in an annual Plum Festival.

Maturing time: minimum 3 months | Calories per 100ml/3½fl oz/scant ½ cup: 255

Makes about 1.5l/52fl oz/6½ cups
750g/1lb 10oz damsons, rinsed
500g/1lb 2oz/2½ cups caster/granulated sugar
750ml/26fl oz/3¼ cups brandy

Prick though the damsons' skins with a sterilized skewer or needle. Put the pierced damsons in a large, sterilized, wide-necked glass bottle or jar (see page 182). Add the sugar and the brandy, then seal and keep in a cool, dark place. Shake the mixture every day until the sugar is completely dissolved, then leave for 3–6 months.

Strain through a sieve/strainer lined with muslin/cheesecloth or a filter and then bottle and store in a cool, dark place, or you can start to drink immediately.

NUTRITION PROFILE (per portion)
1% protein, 0% fat, 98% carbohydrate, 1% fibre

VITAMINS AND MINERALS (percentage of RDA)
Vitamin A 2%, E 2%, C 2%, B1 4%, B5 2%, potassium 6%, calcium 1%, magnesium 1%, iron 1%, zinc 1%, copper 4%

HEALTH BENEFITS
High in antioxidants | helps protect the body against infection

Mountain Berry Liqueur

This liqueur is best made during the autumn after the first frost has brought out the full flavour of ripe rowan berries. Pick them when out on a forest walk, and then enjoy this warming, invigorating liqueur on cold winter nights.

Maturing time: minimum 9 weeks | Calories per 100ml/3½fl oz/scant ½ cup: 290

Makes 750ml/26fl oz/3¼ cups

500g/1lb 2oz rowan berries, rinsed

½ vanilla pod/bean

2 whole cloves

250g/9oz clear honey

500ml/17fl oz/2 cups aquavit (45%)

Put the berries in a sterilized glass bottle or jar (see page 182) with the vanilla pod/bean, cloves, honey and aquavit. Leave to infuse in a cool, dark place for 4–6 weeks, during which time the liquid should become red.

Strain off the berries and the spices through a filter or a sieve/strainer lined with muslin/cheesecloth. Bottle the liqueur and leave for at least 1 month before drinking.

NUTRITION PROFILE (per portion)

3% protein, 7% fat, 85% carbohydrate, 5% fibre

VITAMINS AND MINERALS (percentage of RDA)

Vitamin A 22%, C 49%, iron 7%

HEALTH BENEFITS

Warming and stimulating | benefits digestion and circulation | a traditional remedy for sore throats

GLOSSARY

accessory fruit – also called a pseudofruit, this is a fruit that grows from the thickened end part of the stem (where the flower was) instead of from the ovary, which is the norm. Strawberries and mulberries are examples.

actinidin – a protein-dissolving enzyme found in kiwi fruit. It can aid digestion and act as a blood thinner.

aggregate fruit – a fruit consisting of several merged ovaries, developed from a single flower. Raspberries are an example.

alkaloids – a group of bitter-tasting, natural chemical compounds made by plants, animals and microorganisms. Some are toxic, but others have powerful medicinal actions, including anaesthetic, stimulant, antibacterial, pain-relieving, anti-cancer, antihypertensive and vasodilating effects.

anthocyanins – red, purple or blue pigments found concentrated in the skins of many fruit and vegetables. They have powerful antioxidant and anti-inflammatory properties.

antioxidants – protect cells from damage caused by unstable molecules known as free radicals (see page 227).

arbutin – an antimicrobial and mildly diuretic glycoside (see page 227). It inhibits pigmentation and can be useful in treating urinary tract infections.

berry – in botanical terms, a berry is a fleshy fruit made from a single ovary, with the seeds embedded within it. Grapes and tomatoes are examples. In everyday speech, a berry is any small, juicy, brightly coloured edible fruit with a sweet, tart or sour flavour.

beta-carotene – a bright red-orange, fat-soluble, antioxidant plant pigment and a good, non-toxic source of vitamin A. It promotes healthy eyes and skin, but excess intake may cause the skin to turn orange (though this is usually reversible). Blackberries, cherries, damsons, sea-buckthorn and persimmons contain high levels of beta-carotene.

bioflavonoids – see flavonoids (see page 227).

calyx – the outer covering of a flower bud consisting of individual sepals. The calyx is usually, but not always, green in colour.

carotenoids – a group of antioxidant organic pigments, ranging in colour from pale yellow to bright orange and deep red. They are made during photosynthesis by plants, algae, some bacteria and fungi, and there are over 600 different types including xanthophylls and carotenes.

catechins – slightly bitter, astringent and strongly antioxidant compounds found in many berries. Açai berries have a particularly high content, as does chocolate. They may lessen the severity of allergic reactions and can help protect against strokes, Alzheimer's disease and Parkinson's disease.

chlorophyll – the light-sensitive green pigment in plants and algae responsible for the synthesis of carbohydrates. It can be used therapeutically for detoxification and to promote wound healing.

composite fruit – a fruit that develops from a cluster (or inflorescence) of flowers, each producing single fruits that eventually coalesce and mature into one larger fruit. Mulberries are an example.

compound fruit – a fruit that develops from several ovaries in one or more flowers. Compound fruits can be 'aggregate' or 'composite'.

deciduous – the word means 'falling off', and in botany it is commonly used to describe perennial plants, especially trees and shrubs, that drop their leaves in the autumn.

dioecious – a plant species is said to be dioecious when male and female flowers are found on separate plants. Most plants are bisexual, but some berry species are dioecious, including juniper, mulberry and kiwi fruit.

drupe – a fruit with a single seed contained within a hard stone surrounded by an outer fleshy part. Cherries and damsons are examples.

drupelet – a small drupe, often consisting of several drupelets in a compound fruit. Blackberries and raspberries are examples.

ellagic acid – a natural phenolic antioxidant, produced by many plants, that helps protect body cells from oxidative stress. It is found in high concentrations in berries such as goji, grapes, blackberries, cranberries, raspberries and strawberries.

ellagitannins – a class of antioxidant tannins that are thought to have antibiotic, anti-parasitic and anti-cancer properties. They may also help regulate blood glucose levels.

ethyl gallate – an antioxidant and natural antibiotic found in many plants. It is widely used as an antioxidant food additive (E313).

evergreen – a plant that has foliage throughout the year.

flavonoids – organic plant compounds, also known as bioflavonoids and vitamin P. They are used by plants as chemical messengers, and for UV filtration, pigmentation, nitrogen fixation and metabolism. They are powerful antioxidants with anti-cancer, anti-allergic and antibiotic properties and a reputation for decreasing the rate of memory loss in old age. Examples include lutein, zeaxanthin, carotenoids, catechins, betulinic acid, lycopene and xanthines. Blueberries and strawberries are particularly rich in flavonoids, but most berries have a high flavonoid content.

folate – also known as folic acid or vitamin B9, folate is an essential vitamin that can only be obtained from food (including green leafy vegetables and pulses). Deficiency is associated with many pathologies, particularly anaemia, nerve degeneration and the development of neural tube defects (such as spina bifida) in developing embryos during pregnancy.

free radicals – atoms, molecules or ions that have an uneven number of electrons, making them unstable and highly reactive. This reactivity can cause cell damage if there are too many free radicals present in body tissues, and has the potential to cause serious health problems. Antioxidants are important as they neutralize or 'mop up' excess free radicals in the body.

gallic acid – a phenolic acid found in many plants (often forming a part of tannin molecules). It is an antioxidant that has marked antibiotic and astringent properties.

glucoside – a glycoside derived from glucose, commonly found in plants.

glycoside – plants often store important phytochemicals in the form of glycosides. A glycoside molecule consists of sugar bound to another functional substance, for example, alcohol, anthraquinone, coumarin, saponin or a flavonoid, and it is usually these functional molecules that give plants their medicinal effects.

hydrogen cyanide – also known as prussic acid, hydrogen cyanide is a highly poisonous chemical found in small amounts in bitter almonds and other fruit pits, such as apricot stones, used to make almond-like flavouring.

kaempferol – a natural flavonoid found in many plants and berries. It has antioxidant, anti-inflammatory, antibiotic and anti-allergic properties, and is associated with a reduced risk of cancer and heart disease.

LDL – sometimes referred to as bad cholesterol, LDL (low-density lipoprotein) is one of a group of lipoproteins that the body uses to transport fats around the circulatory system. High blood levels of LDL are associated with cardiovascular problems, such as atherosclerosis, stroke and heart attack.

leucoanthocyanins – also known as proanthocyanins, leucoanthocyanins are colourless flavonoids used by the body in the production of anthocyanins. They are found in many berries including grapes, bilberries, cranberries and blackcurrants.

lignans – a group of antioxidant phytochemicals that includes various phyto-oestrogens.

lutein – a yellow to orange-red carotenoid found in plants, egg yolks and animal fats. It is strongly antioxidant and may protect the eyes from damage resulting from oxidative stress.

lycopene – a bright red carotenoid found in many red fruits and vegetables, especially tomatoes. Considered a powerful antioxidant, it is thought to have potential as an anti-cancer agent. Lycopene is also used as a food colouring (E160d).

melatonin – a hormone found in plants, animals and microbes. It is a powerful antioxidant that protects DNA, stimulates the immune system and helps regulate the sleep-wake cycles. In humans, natural melatonin levels drop with age.

mucilage – a thick, sticky substance produced by plants that can be used to soothe irritation and inflammation of the skin and mucous membranes.

oleic acid – a naturally occurring monounsaturated omega-9 fatty acid found in olive oil and in many other vegetable oils and animal fats.

omega oils, 3 and 6 – omega oils are known as essential fatty acids because they are vital to normal health, but can only be obtained from the diet. Omega-3 oils may help relieve cardiovascular problems such as high blood pressure and varicose veins, but in excess they may increase the risk of bleeding and stroke. They are also thought to reduce the severity of symptoms in ADHD and other autistic spectrum disorders in children, and may enhance mental performance in people of all ages. Omega-6 oils are important for normal hormone and prostaglandin production, but the typical Western diet often contains too much omega 6 in relation to omega 3, which can lead to inflammation-related health problems.

ORAC value (oxygen radical absorbance capacity) – a way of measuring an individual antioxidant's ability to protect tissues from oxidative damage. To date the method has only been used in laboratory settings, and there is as yet no established relationship between ORAC value and health benefit for any particular antioxidant.

oxidative stress – when there are too many free radicals (and other oxidants such as peroxides) in relation to the amount of antioxidants present in body tissues, there is said to be 'oxidative stress'. In this situation, the ability of cells to repair the damage to proteins, fats and DNA is impaired, and oxidative stress is thought to be implicated in many serious chronic health problems, including cancer, cardiovascular problems, neurodegenerative diseases and chronic fatigue syndrome.

parasorbic acid – also known as hexenolactone, parasorbic acid is a potentially toxic chemical found in raw rowan berries. It is active against a broad spectrum of bacteria (gram-positive and gram-negative), and can be used as an antifungal and anti-parasitic agent (particularly against the parasite that causes sleeping sickness). Heating or freezing converts parasorbic acid to sorbic acid, which reduces acidity and increases the sweetness of the berries.

pectin – a polysaccharide found in the cell walls of plants that can be used as a gelling agent. In fruits, pectin is broken down as part of the ripening process, so unripe apples, plums, gooseberries and citrus fruits are the best sources. As pectin is a soluble fibre, eating it as part of a plant-rich diet can help reduce blood cholesterol levels.

perennial – a perennial plant is one that lives for more than two years.

phenols and polyphenols – a group of organic compounds, including tannins, pigments and phyto-hormones, that have antioxidant properties. They are used by plants to make protective UV screens, to provide colour, to deter predators and to protect against infection.

phytic acid – a chemical found mainly in seeds and grains that is used as an antioxidant, as a food preservative (E391) and in chelation therapy (to treat toxic metal poisoning). It is indigestible for humans, but decreases in concentration when seeds and grains are soaked, sprouted or cooked.

phytochemicals – natural compounds in plants that, though not nutrients as such, have a specific biological significance. There are thousands of different phytochemicals in fruit and vegetables with a wide variety of metabolic and medicinal effects. *Phyto* means relating to plants.

phyto-oestrogens – plant-derived oestrogens.

phytosterols – plant-derived steroidal compounds similar to cholesterol, found particularly in plant oils. Phytosterols have been shown to lower blood cholesterol and help maintain normal hormone balance.

pigment – pigments are primarily used by plants for photosynthesis, but also for colour. Examples include chlorophyll, carotenoids, anthocyanins and betalains.

polyphenols – see phenols.

pome – an accessory fruit from the Apple tribe of the Rose family. Rowan berries are pomes.

pseudofruit – see accessory fruit.

quercetin – an antioxidant bioflavonoid with antihistamine, anti-cancer and anti-inflammatory properties.

rapadura sugar – whole organic sugar produced by evaporating sugar cane juice over a low heat without separating out the molasses or adding anti-caking agents.

RDA – the Recommended Daily Allowance of vitamins, minerals and trace elements considered sufficient to maintain good health. It was developed during the Second World War as part of a broader attempt to improve the nutritional health of the population. RDA guidelines are reviewed and changed from time to time and vary from country to country.

resveratrol – a natural phenol produced by plants to help protect them from natural pathogens. It is particularly concentrated in the skins of red grapes and mulberries, and is thought to have very significant effects on human health. Studies suggest that resveratrol can improve stamina, prevent certain cancers, protect against heart and skin diseases and act as an anti-diabetic, anti-inflammatory and antiviral.

riboflavin – another name for vitamin B2, which plays a key role in human energy metabolism. It is orange-red in colour and can be used as a food additive (E101).

rutin – a quercetin compound with antibacterial and antioxidant properites found in abundance in berries such as aronia, cranberry and mulberry. It helps maintain the health of the blood and circulation.

salicylic acid – a phenolic phyto-hormone, originally obtained from willow bark (*Salix*). It can be used to ease aches and pains, reduce fevers and inflammations and as an antiseptic and food preservative. It also has an anti-diabetic effect. Aspirin is made by reacting salicylic acid with acetic anhydride in the presence of an acid catalyst.

scurvy – the medical condition resulting from severe vitamin C deficiency characterized by extreme lethargy and bleeding from mucous membranes.

seitan – also called 'wheat meat', this is made from wheat gluten and has the appearance and texture of cooked meat. It is very high in protein, low in fat and carbohydrate, and rich in iron.

sorbic acid – a natural organic compound, first isolated from rowan berries, that has antimicrobial and antifungal properties and is used as a food preservative (E200–203).

tannin – an astringent, tart and bitter polyphenol, used by plants for growth regulation and as a pesticide. Tannin concentrations fall as plants ripen and they can be used in plant medicine for their astringent, antibacterial, antiviral and antiparasitic properties.

tempeh – a traditional Indonesian soy product made by fermenting whole soybeans and then pressing them into a firm cake. It has an earthy flavour and is an extremely good source of protein, fibre and vitamins.

thiamin (thiamine) – another name for vitamin B1, which is necessary for maintaining the health of the nervous and cardiovascular systems.

tofu – also known as bean curd, tofu is made by coagulating soy milk and pressing the curd into solid blocks. There are many different types available, all with a bland flavour unless spices or soy sauce are added, but all are low in calories and high in protein.

tomatillo – a small green or green-purple berry, which is surrounded by a papery husk and related to the golden berry.

xylitol – a low-calorie sugar that is absorbed by the body slowly. It is used as a sweetener for low-calorie diabetic foods and occurs naturally in various berries and other plant foods.

zeaxanthin or zeathanthin – a common carotenoid pigment that gives colour to paprika peppers, wolfberries, grapes and many other plants. Diet-derived zeaxanthins contribute one of the main carotenoid pigments in the retina of the eye.

INDEX

ACKNOWLEDGEMENTS

Interesting book and web resources consulted during the writing of this book include:

BOOKS

75 Remarkable Fruits for Your Garden, Jack Staub, Gibbs Smith, Layton, Utah, 2007

Bartram's Encyclopedia of Herbal Medicine, Thomas Bartram, Robinson Publishing, London, 1998

Den Grønne Syltebog, 74th edition, Tørsleffs Husmoder Service, Glostrup, 1995

Food as Medicine, Dharma Singh Khalsa, Atria Books, New York, 2003

Growing Fruit, Harry Baker, The Royal Horticultural Society and Mitchell Beazley, London, 1992

Larousse Gastronomique, Octopus Publishing Group, London, 2001

Mit Frugt- og Bærkøkken, Anemette Olesen, Forlaget Hovedland, DK, 2012

Petit Larousse des Plantes qui Guérissent, Gérard Debuigne and François Couplan, Larousse, Paris, 2006

RHS Wisley Experts Gardeners' Advice, The Royal Horticultural Society and Dorling Kindersley, London, 2004

Seasonal Preserves, Joanna Farrow, New Holland Publishers, London, 2010

Superfood Pocketbook, Michael van Straten, Little Books, London, 2008

Superfruits, Paul Gross, McGraw Hill, New York, 2010

The Composition of Foods, McCance and Widdowson, Royal Society of Chemistry, Cambridge, and the Food Standards Agency, London, 2002

The Essential Book of Herbal Medicine, Simon Y. Mills, Arkana, London, 1993

The Neighborhood Forager, Robert K. Henderson, Chelsea Green Publishing Company, Vermont, 2000

The New Oxford Book of Food Plants, J.G. Vaughan and C.A. Geissler, Oxford University Press, Oxford, 1999

The Oxford Book of Health Foods, J.G. Vaughan and P.A. Judd, Oxford University Press, Oxford, 2003

Wild Edible Fruits and Berries, Marjorie Furlong and Virginia Pill, Naturegraph Publishing, Happy Camp, 2003

Acknowledgements

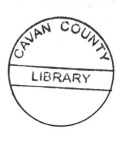

WEBSITES

blackcurrantfoundation.co.uk

britishtomatoes.co.uk

edible wild plant index

food.com

foodreference.com

Harvard Medical School

Kew Gardens

nutritiondata.self.com

MediHerb.com

Plants For A Future

skovdyrkerne.dk

The American Botanical Council

The Royal Horticultural Society

wikipedia.org

The author would like to thank the following people for their help during the writing of this book:

Allan Hartvig

Anders Hartvig

Anette Gundersen

Ann Brit Fogde

Anna

Lille Vildmosecentret

Carolyn Ryden

Cecile Charmetant

Charlotte Charmetant

Den Økologiske Have i Odder

Dominique d'Escaro

Emilie Rose

Erik Buchreitz

Erik Gundersen

Grete Lyngdorf

Hans Knaehus

Helle Buchreitz

Hildur Jackson

Inga Ørnstrup

Jakob Buchreitz

Jennifer Maughan

Karna Maj

Havenyt

Karen Thyregod

Kirsten Hansen

Lauge Buchreitz

Lonnie Nielsen

Michaela Morgan

Nic Rowley

Ole Boi

Paul Charmetant

Peter Firebrace

Raphael Charmetant

Rebecca Woods

Rob Ward

Robert Saxton

Roger Walton

Ry Højskole

Søren Buchreitz

Tara Firebrace

Tessa Hodsdon

Special thanks to Karsten Smith from Restaurant Elverhøj for help with the recipes.

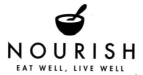

NOURISH
EAT WELL, LIVE WELL

Here at Nourish we're all about wellbeing through food and drink – irresistible dishes with a serious good-for-you factor. If you want to eat and drink delicious things that set you up for the day, suit any special diets, keep you healthy and make the most of the ingredients you have, we've got some great ideas to share with you. Come over to our blog for wholesome recipes and fresh inspiration – **nourishbooks.com**.